Nursing Know-How

Evaluating Heart & Breath Sounds

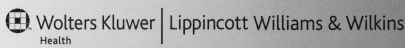

Wolters Kluwer | Lippincott Williams & Wilkins
Health

Philadelphia · Baltimore · New York · London
Buenos Aires · Hong Kong · Sydney · Tokyo

STAFF

Executive Publisher
Judith A. Schilling McCann, RN, MSN

Editorial Director
H. Nancy Holmes

Clinical Director
Joan M. Robinson, RN, MSN

Art Director
Mary Ludwicki

Editorial Project Manager
Sean Webb

Clinical Project Manager
Kathryn Henry, RN, BSN, CCRC

Editor
Catherine E. Harold

Copy Editors
Kimberly Bilotta (supervisor),
Linda Hager, Jeannine Fielding,
Amy Furman, Elizabeth Mooney,
Dorothy P. Terry, Pamela Wingrod

Designers
Arlene Putterman, BJ Crim, Joseph John
Clark (cover design)

Digital Composition Services
Diane Paluba (manager), Joyce Rossi Biletz,
Donna S. Morris

Associate Manufacturing Manager
Beth J. Welsh

Editorial Assistants
Karen J. Kirk, Jeri O'Shea, Linda K. Ruhf

Design Assistant
Kate Zulak

Indexer
Deborah Tourtlotte

The clinical treatments described and recommended in this publication are based on research and consultation with nursing, medical, and legal authorities. To the best of our knowledge, these procedures reflect currently accepted practice. Nevertheless, they can't be considered absolute and universal recommendations. For individual applications, all recommendations must be considered in light of the patient's clinical condition and, before administration of new or infrequently used drugs, in light of the latest package-insert information. The authors and publisher disclaim any responsibility for any adverse effects resulting from the suggested procedures, from any undetected errors, or from the reader's misunderstanding of the text.

NKHEHBS010508

**Library of Congress
Cataloging-in-Publication Data**

Nursing know-how. Evaluating heart & breath sounds.
    p. ; cm.
    Includes bibliographical references and index.
    1. Heart–Sounds–Handbooks, manuals, etc. 2. Lungs–Sounds–Handbooks, manuals, etc. 3. Auscultation–Handbooks, manuals, etc. 4. Nursing diagnosis–Handbooks, manuals, etc. I. Title: Evaluating heart & breath sounds. II. Title: Evaluating heart and breath sounds.
    [DNLM: 1. Heart Auscultation–nursing–Handbooks. 2. Cardiovascular Diseases–nursing–Handbooks. 3. Respiratory Sounds–Handbooks. 4. Respiratory Tract Diseases–nursing–Handbooks. WY 49 N97495 2008]
    RC683.5.A9N87 2008
    616.07'5–dc22
    ISBN-13: 978-0-7817-9203-5 (alk. paper)
    ISBN-10: 0-7817-9203-7 (alk. paper)
    2008005029

Contents

Appendices and index

Contributors and consultants

W. Chad Barefoot, ACNP, MSN
Acute/Critical Care Nurse Practitioner
Abington Pulmonary & Critical Care Associates, Ltd.
Abington (Pa.) Memorial Hospital

Nancy Blumenthal, CRNP, MSN
Senior Nurse Practitioner, Lung Transplant Program
University of Pennsylvania Medical Center
Philadelphia

Wendy Tagan Conroy, APRN,BC, MSN
Nurse Practitioner
Connecticut Valley Hospital
Middletown

Anne W. Davis, RN, PhD
Professor of Nursing
East Central University
Ada, Okla.

Louise Diehl-Oplinger, RN, MSN, APRN,BC, CCRN, NP-C
Nurse Practitioner, Practice Owner
Lehigh Valley Wellness Center
Phillipsburg, N.J.

Nancy J. Gilliam, RN, MS, APN,BC, CRNP
Nurse Practitioner
Amin Heart Associates
Easton, Pa.
Adjunct Clinical Faculty
Warren County Community College
Washington, N.J.

Gary R. Jones, FNP-C, MSN
Nurse Practitioner
St. Johns Heart Care
Joplin, Mo.

Jennifer M. Lee, FNP-C, MSN, CCRN
Nurse Practitioner
Greenville (S.C.) Memorial Hospital – Pulmonary Disease Associates

Nicolette C. Mininni, RN, MEd, CCRN
Advanced Practice Nurse, Critical Care
Mid America Heart Institute
University of Pittsburgh Medical Center, Shadyside

Nancy M. Richards, RN, MSN, CCNS, CCRN
Cardiovascular Surgery Clinical Nurse Specialist
Mid America Heart Institute
Saint Luke's Hospital
Kansas City, Mo.

Patricia Walters, RN, MSN, APN-C, CCRN
Nurse Practitioner, Cardiac Surgery
Hackensack (N.J.) University Medical Center

Part one

Heart sounds

1 Cardiac anatomy and physiology

The cardiovascular system (sometimes called the *circulatory system*) consists of the heart, blood vessels, and lymphatics. A powerful muscular organ, the heart pumps blood to all organs and tissues in the body. The vascular network—comprising the arteries and veins—carries blood throughout the body, keeps the heart filled with blood, and maintains blood pressure. This chapter discusses each part of this critical system.

Heart anatomy

The heart lies in the mediastinum, beneath the sternum and between the lungs and the second and sixth ribs. In most people, the heart lies obliquely, with the right side below and almost in front of the left. Because of its oblique angle, the heart's base (the top of the heart) is located at its upper right, and its pointed apex (the bottom of the heart) is located at its lower left. The apex is the point of maximal impulse, where heart sounds are the loudest.

On average, an adult's heart is about the size of a fist. (See *Dimensions of an average-sized adult heart.*) The heart gradually increases in size from infancy through early adulthood and is usually slightly larger in men than in women. It contains cardiac and smooth muscles.

A sac called the *pericardium* surrounds the heart, and a thin wall (called the septum) divides the heart into right and left sides. Each side is further divided into two chambers (an atrium and a ventricle). The heart also contains four valves (two atrioventricular [AV] and two semilunar valves). (See *Inside a normal heart,* page 4.)

Dimensions of an average-sized adult heart

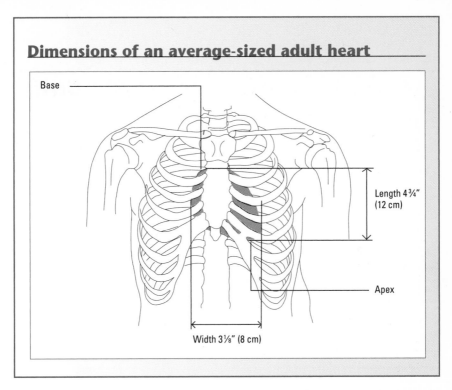

Base

Length 4¾"
(12 cm)

Apex

Width 3⅛" (8 cm)

The pericardium is a two-layer fibroserous sac that surrounds the heart and the roots of the great vessels (those that enter and leave the heart). It consists of the fibrous pericardium and the serous pericardium.

The fibrous pericardium, composed of tough, white fibrous tissue, fits loosely around the heart, protecting it. The serous pericardium, the thin, smooth inner portion of the pericardium, has two layers:

■ The parietal layer lines the inside of the fibrous pericardium.

■ The visceral layer adheres to the surface of the heart.

Between the fibrous and serous pericardium is the pericardial space. This space contains pericardial fluid that lubricates the space and allows the heart to move easily during contraction.

The wall of the heart consists of three layers:

■ The epicardium, the outer layer (and the visceral layer of the serous pericardium), is made up of squamous epithelial cells overlying connective tissue.

■ The myocardium, the middle layer, forms most of the heart wall. It has striated muscle fibers that cause the heart to contract.

Inside a normal heart

The heart contains four chambers (two atria and two ventricles) and four valves (two atrioventricular and two semilunar valves). A network of blood vessels carries blood to and from the heart.

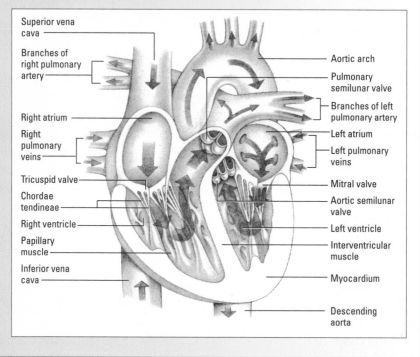

- The endocardium, the heart's inner layer, consists of endothelial tissue with small blood vessels and bundles of smooth muscle.

Chambers

The heart contains four hollow chambers: two atria (the plural form of the word atrium) and two ventricles. The atria, the upper chambers, are separated by the interatrial septum. They receive blood returning to the heart and pump blood into the ventricles. The right atrium receives blood from the superior and inferior venae cavae. The left atrium, which is smaller but has thicker walls than the right atrium, forms the uppermost part of the heart's left border. It receives blood from the two pulmonary veins.

The right and left ventricles, which are separated by the interventricular septum, make up the two lower chambers. The ventricles receive blood from the atria. Composed of highly developed musculature, the ventricles are larger and have thicker walls than the atria.

The right ventricle receives blood from the right atrium and pumps it through the pulmonary arteries to the lungs. The left ventricle, which is larger than the right, receives oxygenated blood from the left atrium and pumps it through the aorta to all other vessels of the body.

Valves

The heart contains four valves: two AV valves and two semilunar valves. The valves allow blood to flow forward through the heart and prevent it from flowing backward. They open and close in response to pressure changes caused by ventricular contraction and blood ejection.

The two AV valves separate the atria from the ventricles. The right AV valve, called the *tricuspid valve,* prevents backflow from the right ventricle into the right atrium. The left AV valve, called the *mitral valve,* prevents backflow from the left ventricle into the left atrium.

One of the two semilunar valves is the pulmonic valve, which prevents backflow from the pulmonary artery into the right ventricle. The other semilunar valve is the aortic valve, which prevents backflow from the aorta into the left ventricle.

The tricuspid valve has three triangular cusps, or leaflets. The mitral valve, also called the *bicuspid valve,* contains two cusps, a large anterior and a smaller posterior. Chordae tendineae (tendinous cords) attach the cusps of the two AV valves to papillary muscles in the ventricles. These cords vary in length and thickness and, in many cases, branch out. The semilunar valves have three cusps that are shaped like half-moons—hence, the name semilunar.

Heart function

The heart's job is to keep blood flowing throughout the circulatory system, delivering oxygen to and removing waste products from the body's cells. The heart actually consists of two separate pumps, one on the right and one on the left.

Specifically, the left side of the heart pumps out oxygenated blood, which the circulatory system delivers to all the body's tissues. The cells take up the oxygen and release carbon dioxide, a waste product.

Pathways of oxygenated and deoxygenated blood

Oxygenated blood travels from the lungs to the left side of the heart, where it's pumped out to the body. Deoxygenated blood returns to the right side of the heart, where it's pumped to the lungs.

OXYGENATED BLOOD PATH

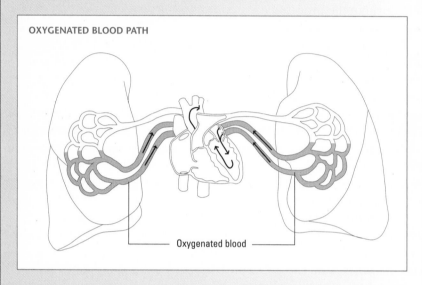

Oxygenated blood

DEOXYGENATED BLOOD PATH

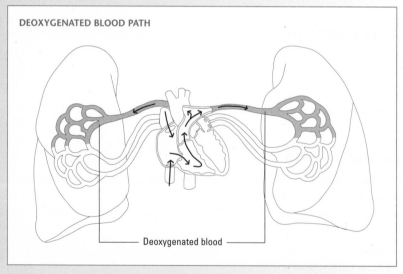

Deoxygenated blood

The circulatory system then carries the deoxygenated blood back to the right side of the heart.

After receiving blood from the systemic circulation, the right side of the heart pumps it to the lungs. There, the blood releases carbon dioxide, which the lungs excrete. The blood also picks up oxygen from the lungs. The oxygenated blood then travels back to the left side of the heart, where the process begins again. (See *Pathways of oxygenated and deoxygenated blood.*)

The average healthy adult heart pumps approximately 5 to 7 L of blood per minute, or 1,500 to 2,000 gallons per day. The heart performs this task continuously throughout a person's life; however, pumping efficiency can change with age.

AGE ALERT *As a normal part of aging, contractile strength declines, making the heart less efficient. In most people, resting cardiac output diminishes 30% to 35% by age 70. In addition, veins dilate and stretch with age, and coronary artery blood flow drops 35% between ages 20 and 60. The aorta becomes more rigid, causing systolic blood pressure to rise disproportionately higher than diastolic pressure, resulting in a widened pulse pressure. Between ages 30 and 80, the left ventricular wall grows 25% thicker from its increased efforts to pump blood. Heart valves also become thicker from fibrotic and sclerotic changes. This thickening can prevent the valves from closing completely, causing systolic murmurs.*

Heart conduction

The heart's conduction system consists of specialized cells and fibers that produce electrical impulses. These electrical impulses discharge automatically, causing the heart muscles to contract and pump blood through the body. The heart's pattern of contraction and relaxation is called the *cardiac cycle.* (See *Cardiac conduction system,* page 8.)

Electrical impulses

The conduction system of the heart contains pacemaker cells that have three unique characteristics:
- automaticity—the ability to generate an electrical impulse automatically
- conductivity—the ability to pass the impulse to the next cell
- contractility—the ability to shorten the fibers in the heart when receiving the impulse.

Cardiac conduction system

Specialized fibers carry electrical impulses through the heart muscle, causing the heart to contract. This illustration shows the elements of the cardiac conduction system.

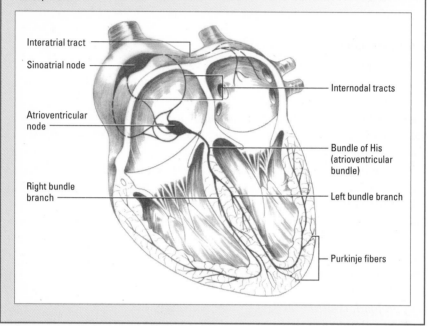

The sinoatrial (SA) node—located on the endocardial surface of the right atrium, just below the entrance to the superior vena cava—is the normal pacemaker of the heart. As such, it generates electrical impulses between 60 and 100 times per minute. The firing of the SA node spreads each impulse throughout the right and left atria, resulting in atrial contraction.

The AV node, located low in the septal wall of the right atrium, receives the impulse from the SA node and slows impulse conduction between the atria and ventricles. This "resistor" node allows time for the contracting atria to fill the ventricles with blood before the lower chambers contract.

From the AV node, the impulse travels to the bundle of His (modified cardiac muscle fibers), branching off to the right and left bundles. Finally, the impulse travels to tiny Purkinje fibers, the distal portions of the left and right bundle branches. These fibers fan across the surface of the ventricles from the endocardium to the myocardium. As the impulse spreads, it instructs the blood-filled ventricles to contract.

The conduction system has two built-in safety mechanisms. If the SA node fails to fire, the AV node generates impulses between 40 and 60 times per minute. If the SA node and the AV node fail, the ventricles can generate their own impulses between 20 and 40 times per minute.

Cardiac cycle

The cardiac cycle is the period from the beginning of one heartbeat to the beginning of the next. (See *Phases of the cardiac cycle,* page 10.) During this cycle, electrical and mechanical events must occur in the proper sequence and to the proper degree to provide adequate blood flow to all body parts. The cardiac cycle has two main events: systole (contraction) and diastole (relaxation).

At the beginning of atrial systole, the atria, which are filled with blood, contract and push blood into the ventricles. After the ventricles fill, ventricular systole occurs and the ventricles contract. Ventricular blood pressure builds until it exceeds the pressures in the pulmonary artery and the aorta. The pressure creates enough force to close the AV valves (mitral and tricuspid) and to open the semilunar valves (pulmonic and aortic). When the semilunar valves open, the ventricles eject blood into the aorta and the pulmonary artery. (See *Understanding preload, contractility, and afterload,* page 11.)

When the ventricles empty and relax, ventricular pressure falls below the pressures in the pulmonary artery and the aorta. At the beginning of diastole, the semilunar valves close to prevent the backflow of blood into the ventricles, and the mitral and tricuspid valves open, allowing blood to flow into the ventricles from the atria. When the ventricles become full, near the end of this phase, the atria contract to send the remaining blood to the ventricles. Then a new cardiac cycle begins as the heart enters systole again.

Cardiac output (CO) refers to the amount of blood the heart pumps in 1 minute. It's equal to the heart rate (HR) multiplied by the stroke volume (SV), the amount of blood ejected with each heartbeat ($CO = HR \times SV$). Stroke volume, in turn, depends on three major factors: preload, contractility, and afterload. To determine SV, use the equation $SV = CO \div HR$.

Phases of the cardiac cycle

The cardiac cycle consists of five phases, as described here.

Isovolumetric ventricular contraction

In response to ventricular depolarization, tension in the ventricles increases. This rise in pressure causes the mitral and tricuspid valves to close. The pulmonic and aortic valves stay closed during this phase.

Ventricular ejection

When ventricular pressure exceeds aortic and pulmonary arterial pressures, the aortic and pulmonic valves open, and the ventricles eject blood.

Isovolumetric relaxation

When ventricular pressure falls below the pressures in the aorta and pulmonary artery, the aortic and pulmonic valves close. All valves are closed during this phase. Atrial diastole occurs as blood fills the atria.

Atrial systole

Known as the *atrial kick,* atrial systole (coinciding with late ventricular diastole) supplies the ventricles with the remaining 30% of the blood for each heartbeat.

Ventricular filling

Atrial pressure exceeds ventricular pressure, which causes the mitral and tricuspid valves to open. Blood then flows passively into the ventricles. About 70% of ventricular filling takes place during this phase.

KNOW-HOW

Understanding preload, contractility, and afterload

Thinking of the heart as a balloon can help you understand the three factors that determine stroke volume.

Preload
Preload is the stretching of muscle fibers in the ventricles. Think of a balloon stretching as air is blown into it. The more air, the greater the stretch. In the heart, this stretching results from blood volume in the ventricles at end-diastole.

Contractility
Contractility refers to the inherent ability of the myocardium to contract. According to *Starling's law,* the more the heart muscles stretch during diastole (preload), the more forcefully they contract during systole. In other words, the more air in the balloon, the greater the stretch, and the farther the balloon will fly when air is let out.

Afterload
Afterload refers to the pressure needed for ventricular muscles to overcome the resistance of higher pressure in the aorta, thus pumping blood out of the heart. *Resistance* is like the knot on the end of the balloon, which the balloon has to work against to get the air out.

Vascular system

The body contains about 60,000 miles of blood vessels that keep blood circulating to and from every functioning cell. (See *Major blood vessels,* page 12.) As blood makes its way through this vascular system, it travels through five distinct types of blood vessels involving three methods of circulation.

Blood vessels

The five types of blood vessels are:
- arteries
- arterioles
- veins
- venules
- capillaries.

Major blood vessels

This illustration shows the body's major arteries and veins.

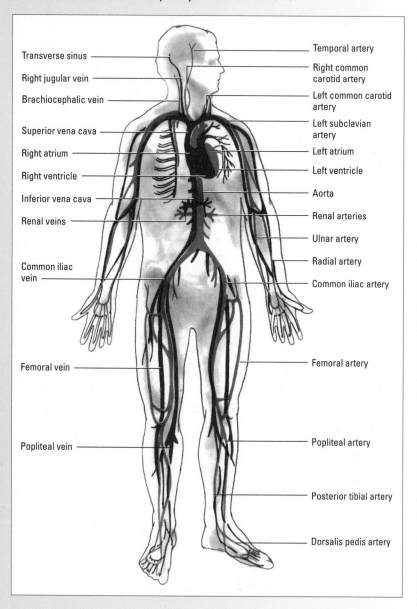

The structure of each type of vessel differs according to its function in the cardiovascular system and the pressure exerted by the volume of blood at various sites within the system.

Arteries and arterioles carry blood away from the heart. Nearly all arteries carry oxygen-rich blood from the heart throughout the rest of the body. The only exception is the pulmonary artery, which carries oxygen-depleted blood from the right ventricle to the lungs. Arteries have thick, muscular walls to accommodate the flow of blood at high speeds and pressures. These walls contain a tough, elastic layer that helps propel blood through the arterial system. Arterioles have thinner walls than arteries. They constrict or dilate to control blood flow to the capillaries.

Veins and venules carry blood toward the heart. Nearly all veins carry oxygen-depleted blood. The only exception is the pulmonary vein, which carries oxygenated blood from the lungs to the left atrium. The walls of veins and venules are thinner than those of arteries and arterioles because of the low blood pressures of venous return to the heart. Veins also have larger diameters and are more pliable than arteries. That pliability allows veins to accommodate variations in blood volume. Veins serve as a large reservoir for circulating blood. They contain valves at periodic intervals to prevent blood from flowing backward.

The exchange of fluid, nutrients, and metabolic wastes between blood and cells occurs in the capillaries. This exchange can occur because capillaries are thin-walled (they're composed of only a single layer of epithelial cells) and highly permeable. About 5% of circulating blood volume at any given moment is contained in the capillary network. Capillaries are connected to the arteries and veins through the arterioles and venules, respectively.

Circulation

Three methods of circulation carry blood throughout the body: pulmonary, systemic, and coronary.

Pulmonary circulation

In pulmonary circulation, blood travels to the lungs to pick up oxygen and release carbon dioxide. As the blood moves from the heart to the lungs and back again, it proceeds as follows:
■ Deoxygenated blood travels from the right ventricle through the pulmonic valve into the pulmonary arteries.

■ Blood passes through progressively smaller arteries and arterioles into the capillaries of the lungs.

■ Blood reaches the alveoli, where it releases carbon dioxide and picks up oxygen.

■ Oxygenated blood then returns via venules and veins to the pulmonary veins, which carry it back to the heart's left atrium.

Systemic circulation

Systemic circulation begins when blood pumped from the left ventricle carries oxygen and other nutrients to body cells. This same circulation also transports waste products for excretion.

The major artery, the aorta, branches into vessels that supply specific organs and areas of the body. As it arches out of the top of the heart and down to the abdomen, three arteries branch off the top of the arch to supply the upper body with blood:

■ The left common carotid artery supplies blood to the brain.

■ The left subclavian artery supplies blood to the arms.

■ The innominate artery supplies blood to the upper chest.

As the aorta descends through the thorax and abdomen, its branches supply the:

■ GI organs

■ genitourinary organs

■ spinal column

■ lower chest

■ abdominal muscles.

Then the aorta divides into the iliac arteries, which further divide into femoral arteries.

As the arteries divide into smaller units, the number of vessels increases dramatically, thereby increasing the area of tissue to which blood flows, also called the *area of perfusion.*

At the end of the arterioles and the beginning of the capillaries, strong sphincters control blood flow into the tissues. These sphincters dilate to permit more flow when needed, close to shunt blood to other areas, or constrict to increase blood pressure.

Although the capillary bed contains the smallest vessels, it supplies blood to the largest number of cells. Capillary pressure is extremely low to allow for the exchange of nutrients, oxygen, and carbon dioxide with body cells. From the capillaries, blood flows into the venules and, eventually, into the veins.

Valves in the veins prevent blood backflow. Pooled blood in each valved segment travels toward the heart by pressure from the moving

Coronary circulation

Coronary circulation includes the arterial system of blood vessels that supply oxygenated blood to the heart and the venous system of blood vessels that remove oxygen-depleted blood from the heart.

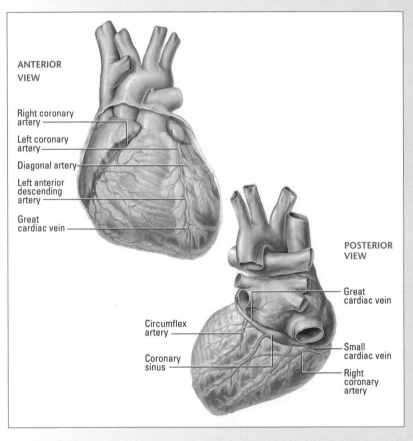

ANTERIOR VIEW

Right coronary artery

Left coronary artery

Diagonal artery

Left anterior descending artery

Great cardiac vein

POSTERIOR VIEW

Circumflex artery

Coronary sinus

Great cardiac vein

Small cardiac vein

Right coronary artery

volume of blood from below. The veins merge until they form two main branches, the superior vena cava and inferior vena cava, which return blood to the right atrium.

Coronary circulation

The heart relies on the coronary arteries and their branches for its supply of oxygenated blood. It depends on the cardiac veins to remove oxygen-depleted blood. (See *Coronary circulation*.)

During left ventricular systole, blood is ejected into the aorta. During diastole, blood flows out of the heart and then through the coronary arteries to nourish the heart muscle.

The right coronary artery supplies blood to the right atrium, part of the left atrium, most of the right ventricle, and the inferior part of the left ventricle. The left coronary artery, which splits into the anterior descending artery and circumflex artery, supplies blood to the left atrium, most of the left ventricle, and most of the interventricular septum.

The cardiac veins lie superficial to the arteries. The largest vein, the coronary sinus, opens into the right atrium. Most of the major cardiac veins empty into the coronary sinus, except for the anterior cardiac veins, which empty into the right atrium.

2 Cardiovascular assessment

A look at cardiovascular assessment

Careful cardiovascular assessment can help to identify and evaluate changes in your patients' cardiac function. Baseline information obtained during assessment helps guide diagnosis, intervention, and follow-up care.

Complete cardiovascular assessment consists of obtaining an accurate, thorough health history and performing a physical examination, including assessing the patient's heart and vascular system. Note, however, that if your patient is in a cardiac crisis, you'll have to rethink your assessment priorities. The patient's condition and the clinical situation dictate what steps you should take.

Obtaining a health history

Begin your cardiovascular assessment by introducing yourself to the patient and explaining what will occur during the health history and physical examination. For the history portion of your assessment, ask about the patient's chief complaint as well as personal and family history of disease. Be sure to document all of your findings.

Chief complaint

Begin the health history by asking the patient why he's seeking medical care. If he has chest pain, ask him to rate the pain on a scale of 1 to 10, in which 1 means that the pain is negligible and 10 means it's the worst pain imaginable. Ask about the pain's:

Key questions for assessing cardiac function

The following questions and statements will help you to assess your patient more accurately:

- Tell me about any feelings of shortness of breath you have. Does a particular body position seem to bring it on? Which one? How long does shortness of breath last? What relieves it?
- Has sudden breathing trouble ever awakened you from sleep? Tell me more about this.
- Do you use more than one pillow at night to help you breathe? If so, how many?
- Do you ever wake up coughing? How often? Have you ever coughed up blood?
- Does your heart ever pound, beat fast, flutter, or skip a beat? If so, when does this happen?
- Do you ever get dizzy or faint? What seems to bring this on?
- Tell me about any swelling in your hands, ankles, or feet. What time of day does this usually occur? Does anything relieve the swelling?
- Have you noticed any changes in color, temperature, or sensation in your legs? If so, which leg? Describe the changes.
- Do you urinate often at night?
- Tell me how you feel while you're doing your daily activities. Have you had to limit your activities or rest often while doing them?

- location
- radiation
- duration
- precipitating factors
- exacerbating factors
- relieving factors.

Also ask the patient if he has other symptoms, such as dizziness, nausea, or sweating.

Let the patient describe his problem in his own words. Avoid leading questions. If the patient isn't in distress, ask questions requiring more than a "yes" or "no" response. (See *Key questions for assessing cardiac function.*)

Vein changes in pregnancy

You might find 4+ pitting edema in the legs of a pregnant patient in her third trimester. Severe edema is common not just in the third trimester but also in pregnant women who stand for long periods. Varicose veins are another common finding in the third trimester.

Other ailments

Patients with cardiovascular problems also commonly complain of:
- headaches
- shortness of breath
- dizziness
- excess fatigue
- unexplained weight changes
- high or low blood pressure
- pain in the limbs (such as leg pain or cramps)
- swelling of the limbs. (See *Vein changes in pregnancy.*)

They may also report peripheral skin changes, such as decreased hair distribution, skin color changes, or a thin, shiny appearance of the skin.

Personal and family history

After you've asked about the patient's chief complaint, inquire about his personal and family medical history, including heart disease, diabetes, and chronic lung, kidney, or liver disease.

 AGE ALERT As you assess a patient, remember that age, sex, and race are essential considerations in identifying the risk of cardiovascular disorders. For example, coronary artery disease most commonly affects white males between ages 40 and 60. Females are also vulnerable to heart disease, especially postmenopausal females and those with diabetes mellitus. Hypertension occurs most often in blacks. Many elderly people have increased systolic blood pressure because of an increase in the rigidity of their blood vessel walls with age. Overall, elderly people have a higher incidence of cardiovascular disease than do younger people.

Also ask the patient about his:
- stress level and coping mechanisms
- current health habits, such as smoking, alcohol intake, caffeine intake, exercise, and dietary intake of fat and sodium

- drug use, including over-the-counter drugs, vitamins, and herbal preparations
- previous surgeries
- environmental or occupational hazards
- activities of daily living.

Performing a physical assessment

Cardiovascular disease affects people of all ages and can take many forms. A consistent, methodical approach to assessment can help you identify abnormalities. As always, the key to accurate assessment is regular practice, which helps to improve technique and efficiency.

Before you begin your physical assessment, you'll need:
- a stethoscope with a bell and a diaphragm
- a blood pressure cuff of appropriate size
- a ruler
- a penlight or other flexible light source.

Also, make sure the room is quiet. Ask the patient to remove all clothing except his underwear and to put on an examination gown. Have the patient lie on his back, with the head of the examination table at a 30- to 45-degree angle, depending on the patient's comfort level and respiratory status. Stand on the patient's right side if you're right-handed or his left side if you're left-handed so you can auscultate more easily.

Assessing the heart

Assessing the heart involves inspection, palpation, percussion, and auscultation.

 KNOW-HOW *To remember the order in which you should perform assessment of the cardiovascular system, just think, "I'll Properly Perform Assessment." (Inspection, Palpation, Percussion, Auscultation)*

Inspection

First, take a moment to assess the patient's general appearance. Is he overly thin? Obese? Alert? Anxious? Next, inspect the patient's precordium (the anterior region of the chest and thorax, including the epigastric area). Note landmarks you can use to describe your findings as well as structures underlying the chest wall. (See *Inspecting and palpating the precordium.*)

Inspecting and palpating the precordium

To inspect and palpate the precordium, locate the six precordial areas described below using the anatomic landmarks named for the underlying structures.

■ Palpate (or inspect) the *sternoclavicular area,* which lies at the top of the sternum at the junction of the clavicles.

■ Move to the *aortic area,* located in the 2nd intercostal space on the right sternal border.

■ Assess the *pulmonary area,* found in the 2nd intercostal space on the left sternal border.

■ Palpate the *right ventricular area* (the point where the 5th rib joins the left sternal border).

■ Then assess the *left ventricular area (apical area),* which falls at the 5th intercostal space at the midclavicular line.

■ Finally, palpate the *epigastric area* at the base of the sternum between the cartilage of the left and right 7th ribs. Avoid pressing on the xiphoid process.

The views below show where to find critical landmarks used in cardiovascular assessment.

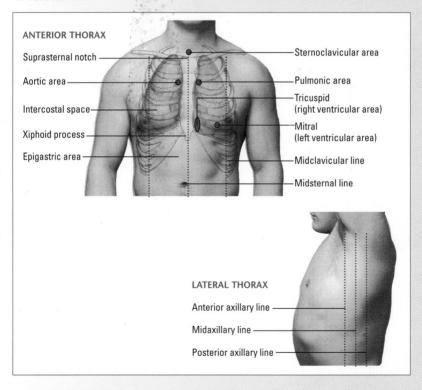

ANTERIOR THORAX

Suprasternal notch — Sternoclavicular area

Aortic area — Pulmonic area

Tricuspid (right ventricular area)

Intercostal space — Mitral (left ventricular area)

Xiphoid process —

Epigastric area — Midclavicular line

Midsternal line

LATERAL THORAX

Anterior axillary line

Midaxillary line

Posterior axillary line

Also look for pulsations, symmetry of movement, retractions, or heaves. A heave is a strong outward thrust of the chest wall that occurs during systole. Note any deviations from the typical chest shape and movement.

Position a light source, such as a flashlight or gooseneck lamp, so that it casts a shadow on the patient's chest. Note the location of the apical pulse. Located in the fifth intercostal space medial to the left midclavicular line, the apical pulse is usually the point of maximal impulse. Because it corresponds to the apex of the heart, the apical pulse indicates how well the left ventricle is working. The apical pulse can be seen in about 50% of adults. You'll notice it more easily in children and in patients with thin chest walls. For obese patients or patients with large breasts, ask them to sit up and lean forward during inspection. This brings the heart closer to the anterior chest wall and makes pulsations more noticeable. To find the apical pulse in a female with large breasts, displace the breasts during the examination.

Palpation

Maintain a gentle touch when you palpate so that you won't obscure pulsations or similar findings. Using the ball of your hand, then your fingertips, palpate over the precordium to find the apical pulse. Note heaves or thrills, fine vibrations that feel like the purring of a cat.

  KNOW-HOW *The apical impulse occurs with the first heart sound and carotid pulsation. To make sure you're feeling the apical pulse and not a muscle spasm or some other pulsation, use one hand to palpate the patient's carotid artery and the other to palpate the apical pulse. Then compare the timing and regularity of the impulses. The apical pulse should roughly coincide with the carotid pulsation. Note the amplitude, intensity, location, and duration of the apical pulse. You should feel a gentle pulsation in an area about ½" to ¾" (1.5 to 2 cm) in diameter.*

The apical pulse may be difficult to palpate in obese and pregnant patients and in patients with thick chest walls. If it's difficult to palpate with the patient lying on his back, have him lie on his left side or sit upright. It may also be helpful to have the patient exhale completely and hold his breath for a few seconds.

Also palpate the sternoclavicular, aortic, pulmonic, tricuspid, and epigastric areas for abnormal pulsations. Normally, you won't feel pulsations in those areas. In a thin patient, though, an aortic arch pulsation in the sternoclavicular area or an abdominal aorta pulsation in the epigastric area may be a normal finding.

Percussion

Although percussion isn't as useful as other methods of cardiac assessment, it may help you locate cardiac borders.

Begin percussing at the anterior axillary line and continue toward the sternum along the fifth intercostal space. The sound changes from resonance to dullness over the left border of the heart, normally at the midclavicular line. The right border of the heart is usually aligned with the sternum and can't be percussed.

Percussion may be difficult in obese patients (because of the fat overlying the chest) or in female patients (because of breast tissue). In this case, a chest X-ray can provide more accurate information about the heart border.

Auscultation

You can learn a great deal about the heart by auscultating for heart sounds. Cardiac auscultation requires a methodical approach and lots of practice. Begin by warming the stethoscope in your hands, and then identify the sites where you'll auscultate: over the four cardiac valves and at Erb's point, the third intercostal space at the left sternal border. Use the bell to hear low-pitched sounds and the diaphragm to hear high-pitched sounds. (See *Sites for heart sounds,* page 24.)

Auscultate for heart sounds with the patient in three positions:
- lying on his back with the head of the bed raised 30 to 45 degrees
- sitting up
- lying on his left side.

Use a zigzag pattern over the precordium. You can start at the apex and work downward or at the base and work upward. Whichever approach you use, be consistent.

Use the diaphragm to listen as you go in one direction; use the bell as you come back in the other direction. Be sure to listen over the entire precordium, not just over the valves.

Note the heart rate and rhythm. Always identify the first and second heart sounds, and then listen for adventitious sounds, such as third and fourth heart sounds, murmurs, and rubs.

Sites for heart sounds

When auscultating for heart sounds, place the stethoscope over the four different sites illustrated here.

Normal heart sounds indicate events in the cardiac cycle, such as the closing
of heart valves, and are reflected to specific areas of the chest wall. Auscultation sites are identified by the names of heart valves but aren't located directly
over the valves. Rather, these sites are located along the pathway blood takes as
it flows through the heart's chambers and valves.

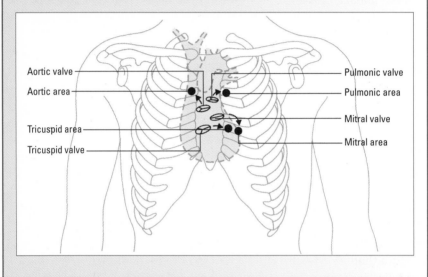

Aortic valve
Aortic area
Tricuspid area
Tricuspid valve

Pulmonic valve
Pulmonic area
Mitral valve
Mitral area

Assessing the vascular system

Assessment of the vascular system is an important part of a full cardiovascular assessment. Your vascular assessment begins with assessing
the patient's vital signs, including temperature, blood pressure, pulse
rate, and respiratory rate. In addition, measure the patient's height and
weight because these measurements help determine cardiovascular
risk factors, drug dosages, and fluid overload. Then proceed with your
examination. Examination of the patient's arms and legs can reveal arterial or venous disorders. Examine the arms when you take vital
signs. Check the legs later during the physical examination, when the
patient is lying on his back. Remember to evaluate leg veins when the
patient is standing.

Inspection

Start your assessment of the vascular system the same way you start an assessment of the cardiac system—by making general observations. Are the arms equal in size? Are the legs symmetrical?

Inspect the skin. It should be warm. Note the color of the skin. Also note how body hair is distributed; it should be distributed symmetrically. Note lesions, scars, clubbing, and edema of the limbs. If the patient is bedridden, check the sacrum for swelling. Examine the fingernails; they should be pink, firm, and free from markings.

Next, make a closer inspection. Start by observing the vessels in the patient's neck. Inspection of these vessels can provide information about blood volume and pressure in the right side of the heart. The carotid artery should appear to have a brisk, localized pulsation. This pulsation doesn't decrease when the patient is upright, when he inhales, or when you palpate the carotid artery. Note whether the pulsations are weak or bounding.

Inspect the jugular veins. The internal jugular vein has a softer, undulating pulsation. Unlike the pulsation of the carotid artery, pulsation of the internal jugular vein changes in response to position, breathing, and palpation. The vein normally protrudes when the patient is lying down and lies flat when he stands.

To check the jugular venous pulse, have the patient lie on his back. Elevate the head of the bed 30 to 45 degrees, and turn the patient's head slightly away from you. Normally, the highest pulsation occurs no more than 1½″ (4 cm) above the sternal notch. Pulsations above that point indicate an elevation in central venous pressure and jugular vein distention.

Palpation

The first step in palpation is to assess the patient's skin temperature, texture, and turgor. Then check capillary refill by assessing the nail beds on the fingers and toes. Refill time should be no more than 3 seconds, or the time it takes to say "capillary refill."

Palpate the patient's arms and legs for temperature and edema. Edema is graded on a four-point scale. If your finger leaves a slight imprint, the edema is recorded as 1+. If your finger leaves a deep imprint that slowly returns to normal, the edema is recorded as 4+.

Also palpate for arterial pulses. (See *Assessing arterial pulses,* pages 26 and 27.) These pulses are pressure waves of blood generated by the pumping action of the heart. All vessels in the arterial system have

Assessing arterial pulses

To assess arterial pulses, use your index and middle fingers. The following illustrations show where to place your fingers to palpate various arterial pulse locations.

Carotid pulse

Lightly place your fingers just medial to the trachea and below the jaw angle. Never palpate both carotid arteries at the same time.

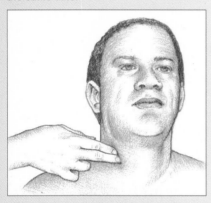

Brachial pulse

Position your fingers medial to the biceps tendon.

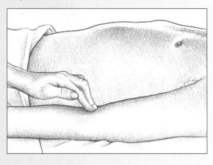

Radial pulse

Apply gentle pressure to the medial and ventral side of the wrist, just below the base of the thumb.

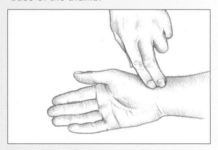

pulsations, but pulsations can be felt only where an artery lies near the skin.

Palpate for arterial pulses by gently pressing with the pads of your index and middle fingers. Start at the top of the patient's body at the temporal artery and work your way down. Check the carotid, brachial, radial, femoral, popliteal, posterior tibial, and dorsalis pedis pulses on each side of the body, comparing pulse volume and symmetry. If you haven't put on gloves for the examination, do so when you palpate the femoral arteries.

Femoral pulse

Press relatively hard at a point inferior to the inguinal ligament. For an obese patient, palpate in the crease of the groin, halfway between the pubic bone and hip bone.

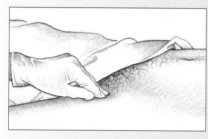

Posterior tibial pulse

Apply pressure behind and slightly below the malleolus of the ankle.

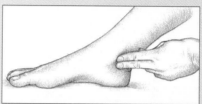

Dorsalis pedis pulse

Place your fingers on the medial dorsum of the foot while the patient points his toes down. The pulse is difficult to palpate here and may seem to be absent in healthy patients.

Popliteal pulse

Press firmly on the popliteal fossa at the back of the knee.

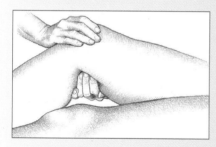

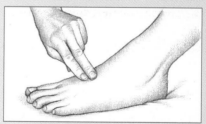

Don't palpate both carotid arteries at the same time or press too firmly. If you do, the patient may faint or become bradycardic.

All pulses should be regular in rhythm and equal in strength. Pulses are graded on the following scale:

- 4+ is bounding.
- 3+ is increased.
- 2+ is normal.
- 1+ is weak.
- 0 is absent.

Performing arterial auscultation

Use these steps when auscultating the carotid, femoral, and popliteal arteries and the abdominal aorta:

■ Ask the patient to hold his breath while you auscultate.

■ Assess the carotid arteries by auscultating with the bell of the stethoscope on both sides of the trachea, as shown here.

■ To evaluate the femoral and popliteal arteries, place the bell of the stethoscope over the pulse sites that you palpated earlier in the assessment.

■ Auscultate the abdominal aorta by listening to the epigastric area.

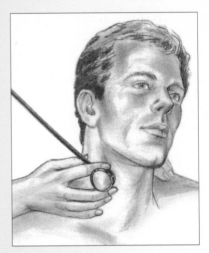

Auscultation

After you palpate, use the bell of the stethoscope to begin auscultation. (See *Performing arterial auscultation*.) Following the palpation sequence, listen over each artery. You shouldn't hear sounds over the carotid arteries. A hum, also called a *bruit*, sounds like buzzing or blowing and could indicate arteriosclerotic plaque formation.

Assess the upper abdomen for abnormal pulsations, which could indicate the presence of an abdominal aortic aneurysm. Finally, auscultate the femoral and popliteal pulses, checking for a bruit or other abnormal sounds.

Interpreting abnormal findings

This section outlines some common abnormal cardiovascular system assessment findings and their causes.

Abnormal skin and hair findings

■ Swelling, or edema, may indicate heart failure or venous insufficiency. It may also be caused by varicosities or thrombophlebitis.

Findings in arterial and venous insufficiency

Assessment findings in patients with arterial insufficiency differ from those in chronic venous insufficiency, as described here.

Arterial insufficiency

In a patient with arterial insufficiency, pulses may be decreased or absent. His skin will be cool, pale, and shiny, and he may have pain in his legs and feet. Ulcerations typically occur in the area around the toes, and the foot usually turns deep red when dependent. Nails may be thick and ridged.

Chronic venous insufficiency

In a patient with chronic venous insufficiency, check for ulcerations around the ankle. Pulses are present but may be difficult to find because of edema. The foot may become cyanotic when dependent.

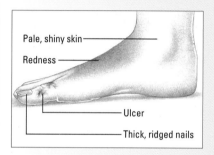

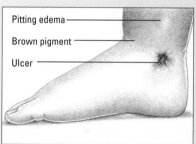

■ Swelling in the lower legs may suggest right-sided heart failure. (See *Findings in arterial and venous insufficiency.*)

■ Ascites and generalized edema may stem from chronic right-sided heart failure.

■ Cyanosis, pallor, and cool or cold skin may indicate poor cardiac output and tissue perfusion.

■ Conditions causing fever or increased cardiac output may make the skin feel warmer than normal.

■ Absence of body hair on the arms or legs may indicate diminished arterial blood flow to those areas.

■ Spongy fingernails indicate clubbing, a sign of chronic hypoxia.

■ Red or brown splinter lines on fingernails suggest bacterial endocarditis.

■ Localized swelling along the path of a vein may indicate compression of a vein in a specific area.

Pulse waveforms

Pulse waveforms can be used to identify the type of an abnormal arterial pulse.

Weak pulse
A weak pulse is characterized by a decreased amplitude with a slower upstroke and downstroke. Possible causes include increased peripheral vascular resistance, which can occur in cold weather or with severe heart failure, and decreased stroke volume, which can occur with hypovolemia or aortic stenosis.

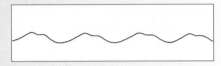

Bounding pulse
A bounding pulse has a sharp upstroke and downstroke with a pointed peak. The amplitude is elevated. Possible causes of a bounding pulse include increased stroke volume, which can occur with aortic insufficiency, or stiffness of arterial walls, which can occur with aging.

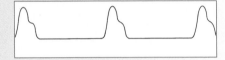

Pulsus alternans
Pulsus alternans is characterized by a regular, alternating pattern of a weak and a strong pulse. This pulse is associated with left-sided heart failure.

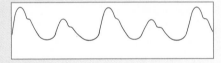

Abnormal pulsations

- A weak arterial pulse may indicate decreased cardiac output or increased peripheral vascular resistance, both of which point to arterial atherosclerotic disease. (See *Pulse waveforms*.)
- A displaced apical impulse may indicate an enlarged left ventricle, which can result from heart failure or hypertension.
- A forceful apical impulse, or one lasting longer than one-third of the cardiac cycle, may point to increased cardiac output.

Pulsus bigeminus
Pulsus bigeminus is similar to pulsus alternans but occurs at irregular intervals. This pulse is caused by premature atrial or ventricular beats.

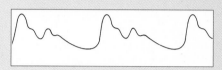

Pulsus paradoxus
Pulsus paradoxus is characterized by increases and decreases in amplitude associated with the respiratory cycle. Marked decreases occur when the patient inhales. Pulsus paradoxus is associated with pericardial tamponade, advanced heart failure, and constrictive pericarditis.

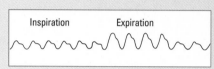

Pulsus biferiens
Pulsus biferiens appears as an initial upstroke, a subsequent downstroke, and then another upstroke during systole. Pulsus biferiens is caused by aortic stenosis and aortic insufficiency.

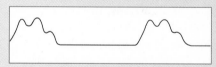

■ If you find a pulsation in the patient's aortic, pulmonic, or tricuspid area, his heart chamber may be enlarged, or he may have valvular disease.

■ Increased cardiac output or an aortic aneurysm may also produce pulsations in the aortic area.

■ A patient with an epigastric pulsation may have early heart failure or an aortic aneurysm.

■ A pulsation in the sternoclavicular area suggests an aortic aneurysm.

■ A patient with anemia, anxiety, increased cardiac output, or a thin chest wall might have slight pulsations to the right and left of the sternum.

■ Strong or bounding pulsations usually occur in patients with conditions that cause increased cardiac output, such as hypertension, hypoxia, anemia, exercise, or anxiety.

■ A heave, a lifting of the chest wall felt during palpation along the left sternal border, may mean right ventricular hypertrophy; over the left ventricular area, a ventricular aneurysm.

■ A thrill, which is a palpable vibration, usually suggests valvular dysfunction.

■ A murmurlike sound of vascular (rather than cardiac) origin is called a *bruit*. If you hear a bruit during arterial auscultation, the patient may have occlusive arterial disease or an arteriovenous fistula. Various high cardiac output conditions—such as anemia, hyperthyroidism, and pheochromocytoma—may also cause bruits. (See *Interpreting cardiovascular assessment findings.*)

Interpreting cardiovascular assessment findings

Clusters of assessment findings may strongly suggest certain cardiovascular disorders. In the table below, the first column shows groups of key signs and symptoms—those that compel the patient to seek medical attention. The second column shows related findings that you may discover during the health history and physical assessment. The third column shows the possible cause of these clustered findings.

KEY SIGNS AND SYMPTOMS	RELATED FINDINGS	POSSIBLE CAUSES
■ Dull or burning chest pain or a feeling of pressure, tightness, or heaviness that builds and fades gradually and may radiate to the abdomen, jaw, teeth, face, or left arm ■ Dyspnea, possibly with a sense of constriction around the larynx or upper trachea ■ Palpitations or skipped beats	■ Family or personal history of coronary artery disease (CAD), atherosclerotic heart disease, stroke, diabetes, gout, or hypertension ■ History of obesity caused by excessive carbohydrate and saturated fat intake; smoking; lack of exercise; stress ■ Male over age 40; postmenopausal female ■ Precipitating factors, such as exertion, stress, hot or cold weather, and emotional turmoil ■ Anxiety, diaphoresis, tachycardia, transient crackles, paradoxical second heart sound (S_2) splitting ■ Blood pressure changes, possibly hypertension, particularly during an episode of chest pain	Angina pectoris

Interpreting cardiovascular assessment findings *(continued)*

KEY SIGNS AND SYMPTOMS	RELATED FINDINGS	POSSIBLE CAUSES
■ Constricting, crushing chest pain like a heavy weight that occurs suddenly, may build to maximum intensity in a few minutes, and usually affects the central and substernal areas but isn't relieved by nitroglycerin ■ Dyspnea, possibly accompanied by orthopnea and cough ■ Fatigue and weakness ■ Palpitations or skipped beats	■ Family or personal history of CAD, stroke, diabetes mellitus, gout, or hypertension ■ History of obesity, smoking, lack of exercise, stress, or angina ■ Anxiety, sense of impending doom ■ Nausea and vomiting ■ Diaphoresis, pallor or cyanosis ■ Tachycardia or bradycardia and weak pulse; arrhythmias ■ Normal or decreased blood pressure ■ Third (S_3) or fourth (S_4) heart sound, pericardial friction rub, or crackles	Acute myocardial infarction
■ Exertional dyspnea ■ Cough ■ Dyspnea at rest (in advanced disease) ■ Orthopnea ■ Paroxysmal nocturnal dyspnea ■ Fatigue on exertion, accompanied by weakness ■ Tachycardia and skipped beats	■ Use of pillows to improve breathing during sleep ■ Wheezing on inspiration and expiration ■ Nocturia ■ Anorexia, progressive weight gain, generalized edema, fatigue ■ Profuse diaphoresis, pallor or cyanosis ■ Frothy white or pink sputum ■ Heaving apical impulse ■ S_3 and S_4, basilar crackles	Left-sided heart failure
■ Dyspnea ■ Fatigue, in severe cases accompanied by weakness and confusion ■ Irregular heartbeat ■ Dependent edema that begins in the ankles and progresses to the legs and genitalia (subsiding at night initially but not later) ■ Weight gain	■ Anorexia, right upper abdominal discomfort, nausea, vomiting ■ History of left-sided heart failure, mitral or pulmonic valve stenosis, tricuspid insufficiency, pulmonary hypertension, or chronic obstructive pulmonary disease ■ Enlarged, tender, pulsating liver ■ Tricuspid insufficiency murmur ■ Ascites, splenomegaly ■ Jugular vein distention, tachycardia, S_3	Acute right-sided heart failure
■ Paroxysmal nocturnal dyspnea accompanied by orthopnea ■ Fatigue ■ Palpitations ■ Possible edema and ascites	■ Signs of heart failure, such as peripheral edema, basilar crackles, dyspnea, and tachycardia ■ Cardiac impulse displaced to the left ■ Systolic murmur, S_3 ■ Orthostatic hypotension	Cardiomyopathies

(continued)

Interpreting cardiovascular assessment findings *(continued)*

KEY SIGNS AND SYMPTOMS	RELATED FINDINGS	POSSIBLE CAUSES
■ Chest pain ■ Dyspnea ■ Fatigue or malaise ■ Weight loss	■ Recent history of acute infection, surgery, instrumentation, dental work, drug abuse, abortion, or transurethral prostatectomy ■ History of rheumatic, congenital, or valvular heart disease ■ Intermittent fever, night sweats, chills ■ Petechiae on conjunctivae and buccal mucosa, splinter hemorrhages beneath nails, pallor or yellow-brown skin ■ Splenomegaly ■ Change in existing heart murmur or development of new murmur ■ Embolization to spleen, kidneys, brain, lungs, or peripheral vasculature ■ Osler's nodes, Roth's spots, and Janeway lesions	Subacute or acute bacterial endocarditis
■ Dyspnea, paroxysmal nocturnal dyspnea ■ Fatigue, usually severe ■ Peripheral edema	■ Female patient ■ History of mitral valve disease ■ Diastolic murmur at lower left sternal border that increases with inspiration, diastolic rumbling ■ Right ventricular lift ■ Ascites, hepatomegaly, jugular vein distention ■ Cyanosis during crying, poor feeding, and poor activity tolerance in a child	Tricuspid stenosis
■ Dyspnea on exertion or at rest ■ Orthopnea ■ Paroxysmal nocturnal dyspnea ■ Hemoptysis ■ Fatigue that worsens as exercise tolerance declines	■ Female patient younger than age 45 ■ Recent bronchitis or upper respiratory tract infection that may worsen symptoms ■ History of rheumatic fever, congenital valve disorder, or tumor (myxoma) ■ Flushed cheeks ■ Lower left parasternal lift or heave ■ Tapping sensation over normal area of apical impulse ■ Middiastolic or presystolic thrill (or both) at apex ■ Small, weak pulse ■ Opening snap	Mitral stenosis
■ Dyspnea on exertion ■ Fatigue ■ Possible peripheral edema	■ History of congenital stenosis or rheumatic heart disease with other congenital heart defects, such as tetralogy of Fallot ■ Jugular vein distention ■ Hepatomegaly ■ Systolic murmur at left sternal border ■ Split S_2 with delayed or absent pulmonary component ■ Cyanosis during crying, poor feeding, and poor activity tolerance in a child	Pulmonic stenosis

Interpreting cardiovascular assessment findings *(continued)*

KEY SIGNS AND SYMPTOMS	RELATED FINDINGS	POSSIBLE CAUSES
■ Dyspnea on exertion ■ Fatigue ■ Syncope ■ Chest pain	■ Aging, history of congenital stenosis, rheumatic fever ■ Systolic murmur of right sternal border ■ Heart failure ■ Pulmonary edema	Aortic stenosis

3 Cardiac auscultation

The cardiovascular system requires more auscultation than any other body system. Gaining the skill needed to detect cardiac abnormalities comes only after lots of practice. To understand auscultation findings, you'll need to use your knowledge of cardiac anatomy and physiology and also apply findings from other parts of the assessment.

Choosing a stethoscope

To perform auscultation, you'll need a stethoscope. The stethoscope picks up the sound of heart vibrations that are transmitted to the chest wall. Some vibrations are easy to hear; others are less distinct. The quality of your stethoscope influences how well you hear subtle differences in sounds. (See *Getting to know your stethoscope*.)

To gain the most from your auscultation assessment, choose a stethoscope with both a diaphragm and a bell. The diaphragm transmits high-pitched sounds more clearly, while the bell transmits low-pitched sounds. You'll also use the bell for pediatric or thin patients, to listen around bandages, and to perform carotid assessment.

A flat, adult-size diaphragm should be about $1\frac{3}{8}"$ (3.5 cm) across. It should also be smooth, thin, and stiff enough to filter out low-frequency sounds. The bell should be about $1"$ (2.5 cm) across and deep enough so that it doesn't fill with skin when you press it against the patient's chest wall. The tubing can range from $10"$ to $15"$ (25 to 38 cm) long, with a diameter of $\frac{1}{8}"$ for shorter tubing and $\frac{3}{16}"$ for longer tubing. The earpieces should fit comfortably inside your ears and cover the external ear canals. Don't use a stethoscope that's too heavy; the excess weight can interfere with your ability to hear sounds accurately. (See *Buying a stethoscope,* page 38.)

Getting to know your stethoscope

Before you begin to auscultate, familiarize yourself with all the parts of your stethoscope. Let's start at the bottom:

■ The *chestpiece,* which rests on the patient's skin during auscultation, consists of a *diaphragm,* a *bell,* or a combination of the two, as shown here.

■ The *stem* is a short metal tube that connects the chestpiece to the tubing. In some stethoscopes, the tubing hides the stem. The stem swivels to open either the diaphragm or the bell for auscultation.

■ Flexible *tubing* connects the stem to the ear tubes. Some stethoscopes have only one tube (single lumen); others have two tubes (double lumen), which may be encased in a single shell.

■ The metal *headset* contains the *binaurals* (ear tubes), *ear tips,* and *tension bar.* To loosen the headset, pull the ear tubes apart; to tighten it, push them together, crossing them as you do so.

■ Fitting snugly into the tubing, two inflexible *binaurals* transmit sound to your ears.

■ The *ear tips,* which come in a variety of sizes and shapes, should fit snugly and comfortably inside your ears.

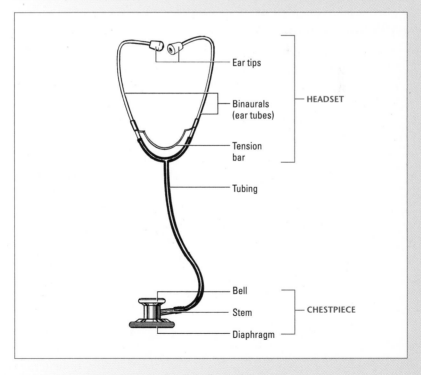

Buying a stethoscope

The first step in buying a stethoscope is to consider the situations in which you'll be using it. For example, do you work in a cardiac unit, a pediatrics facility, or an office setting? Each setting requires different features in a stethoscope. Stethoscopes labeled as cardiology stethoscopes transmit sound more accurately; however, you may not need such an advanced feature. After all, the more features a stethoscope has, the more expensive it will be. Also remember, no matter how sophisticated the stethoscope, the accuracy of the assessment depends on the skill of the person using it.

When making a choice, consider the following variations in chestpieces and tubing.

Chestpiece
■ The chestpiece should have both a diaphragm and a bell.
■ Some stethoscopes have a single-sided chestpiece, which functions like a bell when light pressure is applied and like a diaphragm with firmer pressure.
■ If appropriate, choose an infant chestpiece (¾" diameter) or a pediatric chestpiece (1" diameter).

Tubing
■ Single tubing provides adequate sound for basic assessments.
■ Double tubing, which transmits sound through both tubes, is more sensitive and can yield more accurate auscultation findings. However, the sound of the two tubes rubbing together can be distracting, requiring both you and the patient to remain still.
■ Double-lumen tubing provides the same sound as double tubing, with an added advantage: the outer shell keeps the two tubes from rubbing together, eliminating extraneous noise.
■ Tubing length is mostly a matter of personal preference. Long tubing may dampen sound, although you probably won't notice the decrease. At the same time, long tubing may help you hear low-frequency sounds. When making a choice, consider how close you'll need to be to the patient during auscultation, how you'll carry the stethoscope (such as around your neck or in your pocket), and whether the strain of leaning over to listen with very short tubing would hurt your back.

Auscultation technique

To maximize the effectiveness of auscultation, practice holding the diaphragm and bell correctly. To listen with the diaphragm, either grasp the metal area between the bell and diaphragm with your thumb and index finger or place your fingertips on the rim of the bell. Then press firmly against the chest wall. Apply enough pressure so that a slight indentation remains on the skin after you remove the stethoscope.

When listening with the bell, use a lighter touch. Exerting too much pressure stretches the skin beneath the bell, causing it to act as a diaphragm and filter out low-pitched sounds. To use the bell, grasp the diaphragm's outer edges with your thumb and index finger, and gently rest the bell on the chest wall. Look at the skin around the edges of the bell to make sure you aren't applying too much pressure. If you see signs of indentation, relax the downward pressure.

Don't try to auscultate through clothing or surgical dressings; these items muffle heart sounds or make them inaudible. Instead, open the front of the patient's gown and drape him appropriately to limit the area exposed during auscultation. Make sure that the patient stays warm; muscle movement from shivering can interfere with your ability to hear sounds clearly.

Also, remember to hold the chestpiece so that the tubing doesn't touch you or the patient. Rubbing against the tube can create sounds that interfere with auscultation.

Before you begin auscultation, explain the procedure to the patient. Tell him to breathe normally, inhaling through his nose and exhaling through his mouth. As you prepare to perform cardiac auscultation, make sure the room remains as quiet as possible. If the patient has special equipment, such as oxygen or a suction device, perform auscultation with the equipment turned off, if possible.

Have the patient lie on his back for the first part of the assessment. You may raise the head of the bed slightly if it makes the patient more comfortable. Stand on the patient's right side if you're right-handed and on his left side if you're left-handed so you can manipulate the stethoscope with your dominant hand.

Performing the assessment

To perform the assessment, first identify the sites where you'll auscultate: over the four heart valves and at Erb's point. (See *Auscultatory sequence,* page 40.) When you're ready to auscultate, warm the stetho-

Auscultatory sequence

When auscultating for heart sounds, place the stethoscope over the four valve sites and Erb's point. Follow the same auscultation sequence during every cardiovascular assessment:

■ First, place the stethoscope in the 2nd intercostal space along the right sternal border, as shown. In the aortic area, blood moves from the left ventricle during systole, crossing the aortic valve and flowing through the aortic arch.

■ Then move to the pulmonic area, located in the 2nd intercostal space at the left sternal border. In the pulmonic area, blood ejected from the right ventricle during systole crosses the pulmonic valve and flows through the main pulmonary artery.

■ Next, listen at Erb's point, located in the 3rd intercostal space at the left sternal border. At Erb's point, you'll hear aortic and pulmonic sounds.

■ At the fourth auscultation site, listen over the tricuspid area, which lies in the 5th intercostal space along the left sternal border. In the tricuspid area, sounds reflect blood movement from the right atrium across the tricuspid valve, filling the right ventricle during diastole.

■ Finally, listen in the mitral area, located in the 5th intercostal space near the midclavicular line. (If the patient's heart is enlarged, the mitral area may be closer to the anterior axillary line.) In the mitral (apical) area, sounds represent blood flow across the mitral valve and left ventricular filling during diastole.

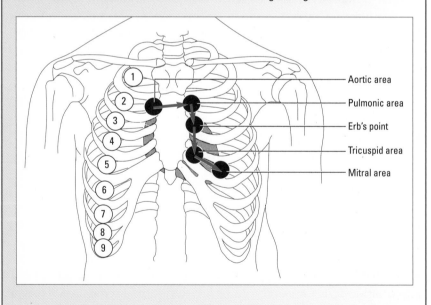

scope between your hands. Remember to listen first with the diaphragm and then with the bell. Listen through several cardiac cycles to become accustomed to the sound, concentrating to hear any subtle changes.

To begin, use the diaphragm, and auscultate at the aortic area where the second heart sound (S_2) is loudest. S_2 is best heard at the base of the heart at the end of ventricular systole. This sound corresponds to closure of the pulmonic and aortic valves and usually is described as sounding like "dub." It's a shorter, higher-pitched, louder sound than the first heart sound (S_1). When the pulmonic valve closes later than the aortic valve during inspiration, you'll hear a split S_2.

From the base of the heart, move to the pulmonic area, then to Erb's point, and then down to the tricuspid area. Next, move to the mitral area, where S_1 is loudest. S_1 is best heard at the apex of the heart. This sound corresponds to closure of the mitral and tricuspid valves and usually is described as sounding like "lub." Low-pitched and dull, S_1 occurs at the beginning of ventricular systole. It may be split if the mitral valve closes just before the tricuspid valve.

Next, listen over the point of maximal impulse, which is usually found in the mitral area. To locate this point, have the patient shift slightly onto his left side into a left lateral decubitus position. This brings the apex of the heart closer to the chest wall. Look closely at the chest wall for pulsations. Then use your fingertips to feel for the pulsation (the apical pulse) between the fourth and sixth intercostal spaces, near the left midclavicular line. Listen here first with the diaphragm and then with the bell.

While performing your assessment, keep in mind that heart valves transmit sound to specific areas of the precordium, not just to specific points. Because these areas overlap each other, focusing on the key sites discussed earlier can help you identify the sounds for each valve. However, in certain instances, such as if the patient has an enlarged heart, you'll need to broaden the area you auscultate. (See *Alternate auscultation areas,* pages 42 and 43.)

After you've completed the auscultatory sequence with the patient lying down, have him sit up, if possible, while you complete the sequence a second time.

Enhancing auscultation findings

Auscultation of heart sounds can be difficult. Even with a stethoscope, the amount of tissue between the source of the sound and the outer

Alternate auscultation areas

When a patient's heart is enlarged, heart sounds extend beyond the traditional auscultation sites. In these instances, broaden your auscultation assessment to include the areas shown in this illustration.

After you've completed your traditional auscultatory sequence, auscultate the alternative areas starting at the apex and working your way up:

■ First, place the stethoscope in the left ventricular area, which is located from the 2nd to the 5th intercostal space, and from the left sternal border to the left midclavicular line. This area increases in all directions if the patient has an enlarged left ventricle. Mitral and aortic murmurs and murmurs in hypertrophic obstructive cardiomyopathy are best heard here.

■ Next, listen at the right ventricular area, located between the 2nd and 5th intercostal spaces over the sternum. If the patient has a severely enlarged right ventricle, the area may extend to the point of maximal impulse. A right ventricular S_3 or S_4 and murmurs from tricuspid stenosis or insufficiency are heard here.

■ Then move to the right atrial area, located along the right sternal border between the 3rd and 5th intercostal spaces. If the patient's right atrium is severely enlarged, this area may extend beyond the right midclavicular line. This area is where the murmur from tricuspid insufficiency is heard best.

■ Next, listen at the left atrial area, located along the left sternal border, between the 2nd and 4th intercostal spaces. Listen here for the murmur resulting from mitral insufficiency.

chest wall can affect which sounds you hear. Fat, muscle, and air tend to reduce sound transmission. If a patient is obese, has a muscular chest wall, or has hyperinflated lungs, the sounds may seem distant and difficult to hear.

If heart sounds seem distant, try placing the patient in an alternate position, which may enhance heart sound auscultation. (See *Alternate auscultation positions,* page 44.)

If placing the patient in an alternate position doesn't amplify heart sounds, methods that change the flow of blood to the heart may help. For example, try auscultating while the patient stands, squats, holds his breath, or raises his legs while lying on his back. Another common technique is to have the patient cough several times or perform Valsalva's maneuver. Keep in mind that Valsalva's maneuver amplifies only systolic murmurs. In other instances, it can interfere with your auscultation efforts.

■ Then move to the pulmonic area, located between the 2nd and 3rd intercostal spaces near the left side of the sternum. Listen here for murmurs from pulmonic stenosis and insufficiency and patent ductus arteriosus.

■ Finally, listen in the aortic area, located from the right 2nd intercostal space to the apex of the heart. This is where you'll hear murmurs from aortic stenosis and insufficiency.

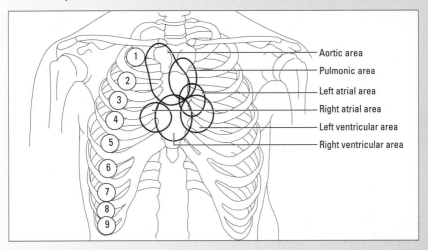

Another method to enhance heart sounds is to have the patient take deep breaths. This slows the patient's respiratory rate, making it easier for you to differentiate between sounds heard during inspiration (reflecting events in the right side of the heart) and expiration (reflecting events occurring in the left side of the heart). Tell the patient that you'll raise your hand when you want him to inhale and that you'll lower your hand when you want him to exhale. Make sure, however, that the patient takes regular, even breaths. Breath holding could inadvertently trigger Valsalva's maneuver, which may alter auscultation findings.

Some patients—such as critically ill patients, elderly patients, children, and patients who don't speak English—present special challenges to the assessment process. (See *Considerations in special populations,* pages 45 and 46.)

Alternate auscultation positions

If heart sounds seem faint or undetectable, you may have to reposition the patient. Alternate positioning may enhance sounds or make them seem louder by bringing the heart closer to the chest's surface. Common alternate positions include a seated, forward-leaning position and the left lateral decubitus position. If these positions don't amplify heart sounds, try auscultating with the patient standing or squatting.

Forward-leaning position

Use the forward-leaning position when listening for high-pitched sounds related to semilunar valve problems, such as aortic and pulmonic valve murmurs. After helping the patient into this position, place the stethoscope's diaphragm over the aortic and pulmonic areas at the right and left second intercostal space.

Left lateral decubitus position

The left lateral decubitus position proves especially helpful when listening for low-pitched sounds related to atrioventricular valve problems, such as mitral valve murmurs and extra heart sounds. After helping the patient into this position, place the stethoscope's bell over the apical area.

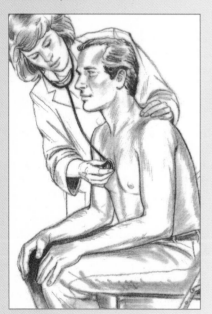

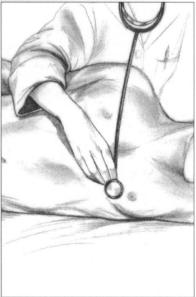

Considerations in special populations

When assessing a patient who is critically ill, elderly, very young, or doesn't speak English, you may need to adjust your usual auscultation process. Using these tips can help the assessment process proceed smoothly.

Critically ill patient

■ Ask for assistance to position the patient properly, especially if he has a ventilator, an intra-aortic balloon pump (IABP), or a Swan-Ganz catheter.

■ Place a patient with left-sided heart failure in the left lateral position. This will bring the heart closer to the chest wall and make the point of maximal impulse easier to locate.

■ To accentuate mitral and tricuspid murmurs, place the patient in a recumbent position.

■ To amplify extraneous heart sounds (such as S_3 and S_4), place the patient in a left semilateral position.

■ To amplify the sound of the tricuspid valve opening, have the patient sit up.

■ If the patient has an IABP, briefly pause the balloon if the patient's condition allows. This will allow you to hear the patient's heart sounds without balloon assistance.

Elderly patient

■ Take into account that degenerative bony prominences can shift cardiac anatomy downward or laterally.

■ Keep in mind that age-related murmurs typically result from incompetent valves.

■ Have the patient sit up and lean forward to accentuate murmurs from aortic or pulmonic regurgitation.

■ Keep in mind that a patient with a memory disorder may become frightened or defensive if you lift his clothing for an assessment. Take time to orient him before you begin.

Pediatric patient

■ Be sure to use an appropriate-size stethoscope. Most stethoscopes have an adapter for a smaller diaphragm.

■ Keep in mind that murmurs in children typically result from ventricular septal defects, patent ductus arteriosus, atrial septal defects, or mitral valve prolapse. Most of these murmurs are harmless and resolve over time.

■ Take into account that exercise, crying, fever, and position changes can accentuate murmurs.

(continued)

Considerations in special populations *(continued)*

Non–English-speaking patient

- Approach the patient in a non-threatening manner.
- Use an interpreter, if possible.
- Demonstrate the assessment process on yourself before assessing the patient.
- Use drawings to enhance your explanation, if appropriate.
- Try to have the patient acknowledge his understanding before you begin.

4 Heart sound origins

The heart sounds you hear through the stethoscope during auscultation are generated by movements of heart walls, valves, and blood contents in response to pressure and volume changes during the heart's rhythmic contractions. These contractions result from electrical activity inside the heart that can be recorded and used to monitor a patient's condition and to guide diagnosis and treatment.

Basic heart sounds

You may hear up to four distinct heart sounds, all of which are described in more detail in chapters 5 and 6:

- The first sound, S_1, occurs at the beginning of systole. It sounds like "lub."
- The second sound, S_2, is produced by closure of the aortic and pulmonary valves. It sounds like "dub."
- The third sound, S_3, is produced by the vibration that occurs when the ventricular walls are suddenly distended by the rush of blood from the heart's atria.
- The fourth sound, S_4, is produced by atrial contraction and ventricular filling.

Normally, however, the heart produces just two basic sounds: S_1 and S_2. **(SOUND 1)** S_1 is heard at the beginning of systole. It's generated by closure of the atrioventricular (AV) valves—the mitral and tricuspid valves. This sound is also associated with increased pressure in the ventricles that causes the moving valve leaflets and cord structures (the chordae tendineae) to slow down. (See *Visualizing the valves producing S_1*, page 48.)

Visualizing the valves producing S₁

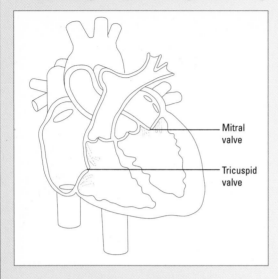

The first heart sound (S₁) is produced by closure of the mitral and tricuspid valves (shown here) and by vibration of the ventricle walls caused by increasing pressure.

Mitral valve

Tricuspid valve

S_2 occurs at the end of systole, when ventricular pressure falls rapidly, causing a slight backflow of blood from the aorta and pulmonary artery. This decrease in ventricular pressure, temporary backflow of blood, and recoiling events cause the aortic and pulmonic valves to close. Vibrations caused by these events produce S_2, which marks the end of ventricular systole. **(SOUND 1)** (See *Visualizing the valves producing S_2.*)

Heart sound characteristics

Every heart sound has six different characteristics that you should assess during auscultation:
- location
- intensity
- duration
- pitch
- quality
- timing.

If you keep these characteristics in mind each time you auscultate, your assessment of heart sounds will be complete, and you'll be able to provide accurate and complete documentation. Also, because these

Visualizing the valves producing S₂

The second heart sound (S₂) is produced by closure of the pulmonic and aortic valves (shown here).

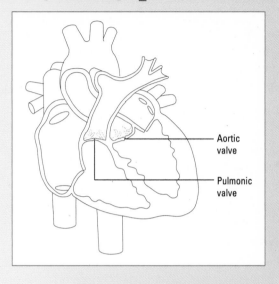

Aortic valve

Pulmonic valve

terms are used universally, all health care professionals will be able to understand your auscultation findings.

Location

A sound's location is the anatomic area on the patient's chest wall where the sound is heard best. Bony structures and landmarks, such as the right and left midclavicular lines, are used to describe the exact location. For example, you might document that S_1 was heard best over the mitral area.

Intensity

Intensity refers to the loudness of the heart sound during auscultation. Usually, intensity is a somewhat subjective assessment based on experience. However, when abnormalities are present, intensity can be determined electronically using a phonocardiogram (PCG). A PCG measures and records the amplitude of the sound's vibrations and allows comparison of auscultated sounds to the heart's recorded electrical activity.

Keep in mind that heart sound intensity is related to the pressures generated and the blood flow velocity inside the heart. It's also related to the patient's size, body build, and chest configuration. For example, a slender patient has a thinner chest wall, which allows sounds to be transmitted more easily than they would be through an obese patient's chest wall. (If a sound is transmitted more easily, the loudness, or intensity, of the heart sound is heard without interference.) What's more, certain interferences, such as pericardial fluid or the lung tissue of a patient with emphysema, can also diminish the amplitude of heart sounds.

Duration

Duration refers to the length of time you hear the heart sound; it can be described as either short or long. Remember, heart sounds are brief vibrations that mark the beginning and end of systole. A sound's duration affects whether you hear it as a click, a snap, or a murmur. For example, murmurs are longer vibrations that are usually caused by blood flow during systole or diastole.

Pitch

The pitch of a heart sound is determined by the frequency of its vibrations. High-frequency sounds (like the notes of a piccolo) are best heard with the diaphragm of the stethoscope; low-frequency sounds (like the notes of a tuba) are best heard with the bell of the stethoscope.

Quality

The quality of a heart sound refers to the type of noise produced. It's determined by the combination of its frequencies. Such words as *sharp, dull, booming, machinelike, rumbling, snapping, blowing, harsh,* and *musical* can be used to describe the quality of heart sounds.

Timing

The timing of a heart sound refers to when you hear it during the cardiac cycle—that is, during systole or diastole.

Depolarization and repolarization

The heart can't pump unless an electrical stimulus occurs first. As electrical impulses are transmitted, cardiac cells go through cycles of depolarization and repolarization. This sequential and rhythmic process is referred to as the heart's electrical activity. Electrical activity occurs at the cellular level in every contractile cell of the myocardium. (See *Understanding the depolarization-repolarization cycle.*)

Understanding the depolarization-repolarization cycle

This illustration can help you understand events that occur during the depolarization-repolarization cycle.

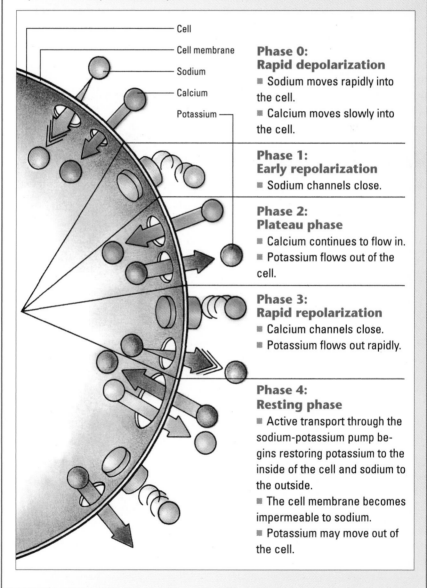

Cell
Cell membrane
Sodium
Calcium
Potassium

Phase 0:
Rapid depolarization
- Sodium moves rapidly into the cell.
- Calcium moves slowly into the cell.

Phase 1:
Early repolarization
- Sodium channels close.

Phase 2:
Plateau phase
- Calcium continues to flow in.
- Potassium flows out of the cell.

Phase 3:
Rapid repolarization
- Calcium channels close.
- Potassium flows out rapidly.

Phase 4:
Resting phase
- Active transport through the sodium-potassium pump begins restoring potassium to the inside of the cell and sodium to the outside.
- The cell membrane becomes impermeable to sodium.
- Potassium may move out of the cell.

Depolarization

Initially, the contractile cardiac cells are polarized (in a resting state). Depolarization begins when the cell membranes become permeable and sodium ions flow into the cell.

Repolarization

When a cell is fully depolarized, it returns to its resting state. This is known as repolarization. Repolarization begins when calcium ions move into the cell and potassium ions begin to move out of the cell. Then, the sodium-potassium pump forces accumulated intracellular sodium and calcium ions out of the cell while the lost potassium is restored to the cell, completing repolarization. The cell is polarized to its original ionic state, and the myocardium relaxes.

Recording heart sounds

Heart sounds are produced by mechanical events that occur in response to an electrical impulse originating in the sinoatrial (SA) node. This electrical impulse travels through the myocardium, activating the atria and ventricles, and can be depicted using an electrocardiogram (ECG). An ECG reflects all of the electrical activity (the depolarization-repolarization cycle) and documents the timing and amplitude of the heart's electrical activity from the atria to the ventricles. (See *The ECG waveform.*)

An ECG represents only electrical activity, not actual pumping of the heart. It's a valuable diagnostic tool that's now a routine part of every cardiovascular evaluation and should be included in the patient's chart.

ECGs help identify primary conduction abnormalities, arrhythmias, cardiac hypertrophy, pericarditis, electrolyte imbalances, and the site and extent of myocardial infarction.

Components of the ECG

The first wave in an ECG occurs when the SA node fires and the impulse spreads through the atria. The P wave, part of the ECG waveform, represents atrial depolarization. Atrial contraction is stimulated by, and closely follows, atrial depolarization.

The ECG waveform

This illustration shows the components of a normal electrocardiogram (ECG) waveform.

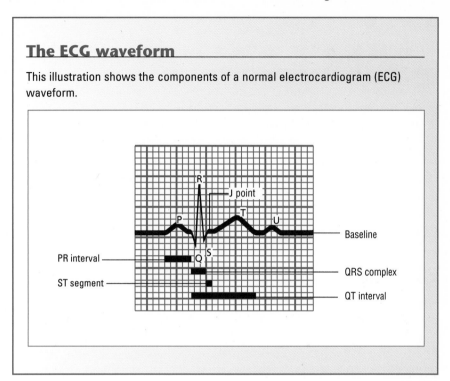

After the P wave, electrical depolarization of the ventricles occurs, producing the QRS complex. Atrial repolarization isn't seen in the ECG because it's hidden in the PR segment and the QRS complex.

Next, during ventricular repolarization, the ventricles relax. This is represented by the T wave on the ECG.

The impulse travels through the AV node, the bundle of His, the bundle branches, and the Purkinje fibers before the ventricles contract. The time between atrial depolarization and ventricular depolarization is recorded on the ECG as the PR interval. It begins at the onset of the P wave and lasts until the onset of the QRS complex. The PR interval correlates with the time interval between atrial contraction and ventricular contraction.

S_1 and S_2 directly correlate with a patient's ECG. S_1 normally occurs just after the QRS complex, and S_2 occurs at the end of the T wave. (See *Finding S_1 and S_2 on the ECG,* page 54.)

Finding S₁ and S₂ on the ECG

The first heart sound (S_1) and the second heart sound (S_2) directly correlate with a patient's electrocardiogram (ECG). S_1 occurs just after the QRS complex, and S_2 occurs at the end of the T wave, as shown here.

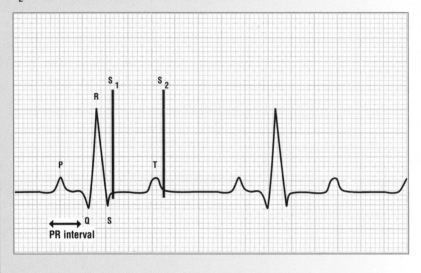

Documenting heart sounds

Each heart sound must be thoroughly documented. By including information about each of the six heart sound characteristics, you can precisely describe every heart sound, whether normal or abnormal. You can document what you heard, where you heard it, how you heard it, and when you heard it. Information about your patient's history can also be a valuable part of heart sound documentation. Consider documenting:

- family history of murmurs or other abnormal heart sounds
- other symptoms present, such as cyanosis, distended neck veins, and abnormal breath sounds.

Although a PCG is one method of graphically representing and documenting heart sounds, it isn't routinely used for every patient; moreover, it requires expensive equipment. Therefore, describing the location, intensity, duration, pitch, quality, and timing is a more practical method of documenting heart sounds. Complete documentation provides other health care professionals with invaluable information that may help them recognize subtle changes in the patient's heart sounds.

5 S_1 and S_2 heart sounds

A heart that's functioning normally produces two basic heart sounds: S_1 and S_2. S_1 results from the closing of the mitral and tricuspid valves. It marks the beginning of systole and is the lub of the lub-dub sequence. S_2 results from the closing of the pulmonic and aortic valves. It marks the end of systole and the beginning of diastole and is the dub of the lub-dub sequence. Becoming familiar with normal heart sounds will help you note variations or abnormal heart sounds.

First heart sound

S_1 is produced by three actions:
- movement of blood in the ventricles
- cardiac vibrations from ventricle walls
- closing of the mitral and tricuspid valves. **(SOUND 2)**

Occasionally, you may hear two components of S_1. Expiration makes them easier to hear. **(SOUND 3)** The first component, known as M_1, stems from closure of the mitral valve; the second component, known as T_1, stems from closure of the tricuspid valve. (See *Valves involved in S_1.*)

The mitral and tricuspid valves close at the beginning of ventricular systole, with the mitral valve usually closing slightly before the tricuspid valve. Because M_1 and T_1 are separated by 20 milliseconds or less, they usually are heard as a single sound, called S_1. (See *Auscultating for S_1, M_1, and T_1.*)

Valves involved in S₁

The valves involved in the first heart sound (S_1) are the tricuspid and mitral valves. S_1 is also caused by the movement of blood in the ventricles and the subsequent vibration of ventricle walls.

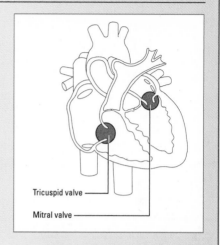

Tricuspid valve

Mitral valve

Auscultating for S₁, M₁, and T₁

To listen to the mitral component (M_1) of the first heart sound (S_1), place your stethoscope over the mitral area, which is located in the 5th intercostal space at the midclavicular line. To hear the tricuspid component (T_1), if it's audible, place your stethoscope over the tricuspid area, located between the 4th and 5th intercostal spaces at the left lower sternal border.

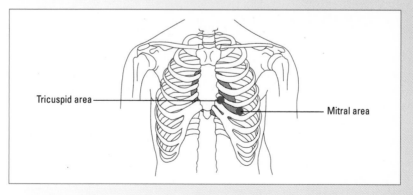

Tricuspid area

Mitral area

Characteristics of S₁

S_1 is usually heard best near the heart's apex over the mitral area at the lower left sternal border. Characteristics of this sound include:
- intensity directly related to the force of ventricular contraction and the PR interval on the electrocardiogram (ECG)
- shorter PR intervals, causing the mitral and tricuspid leaflets to open more widely at the onset of ventricular contraction
- slower heart rate that produces more intense vibrations when the leaflets close, causing a louder S_1
- longer duration than S_2
- high pitch that's heard best with the diaphragm of the stethoscope
- timing that coincides with the beginning of ventricular systole and a palpable carotid pulse **(SOUND 2)**
- S_1 occurring just after the QRS complex in the ECG waveform. (See *S₁ and normal S₁ split on PCG and ECG*.)

> **KNOW-HOW** *Here are some tips to help hear S₁ sounds accurately:*
> - *Auscultate for heart sounds with the patient in the left lateral decubitus, supine, and seated positions. For S₁, alternate using the diaphragm and bell of your stethoscope.*
> - *If S₁ is difficult to identify, palpate for the carotid pulse while auscultating. S₁ will occur just before you feel the carotid pulse. Also, S₁ can be enhanced by sympathetic stimulation, such as that provided by a brief period of exercise.*
> - *For M₁ and T₁, auscultating during expiration may make the sounds more audible.*

Normal S₁ split

As you move the stethoscope from the mitral area toward the tricuspid area, without losing track of S_1, the M_1 and T_1 components of S_1 may become evident. T_1 trails M_1 slightly and is softer; it's heard best near the left sternal border. The timing of M_1 and T_1 with the QRS complex remains the same. The characteristics of the normally split S_1 into M_1 and T_1 are the same. **(SOUND 3)**

Abnormal S₁ split

The normal M_1–T_1 split heard over the tricuspid area widens when electrical activation and contraction of the right ventricle are delayed. Such a delay causes delayed closure of the tricuspid valve, thus widening the interval between M_1 and T_1. **(SOUND 4)**

S₁ and normal S₁ split on PCG and ECG

The first heart sound (S₁) occurs immediately after the QRS complex, as shown below.

PHONOCARDIOGRAM (PCG) AND ELECTROCARDIOGRAM (ECG) SHOWING S₁

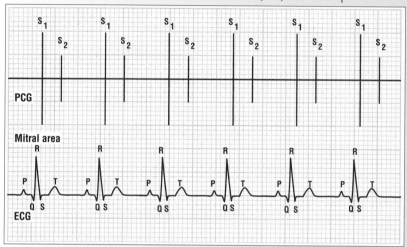

Split sound

In a normal S₁ split, the mitral (M₁) and tricuspid (T₁) components have the same timing as S₁. M₁ occurs slightly before T₁. The second heart sound (S₂) occurs immediately after the T wave.

PCG AND ECG SHOWING NORMAL S₁ SPLIT

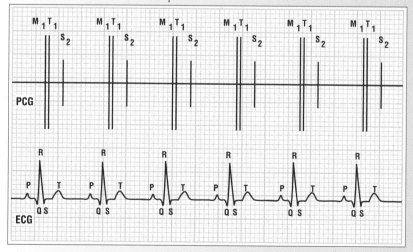

Auscultating for abnormal S₁ split

To auscultate for an abnormal first heart sound (S_1) split, place the stethoscope over the tricuspid area. You may hear a slight delay in the tricuspid component (T_1).

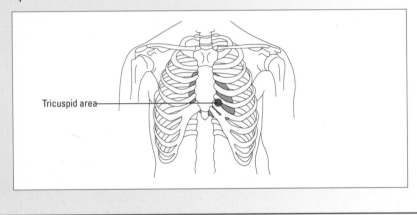

Tricuspid area

The widened interval between M_1 and T_1 is an abnormal S_1 split that may be referred to as a widened S_1 split. Widened S_1 splits are associated with complete right bundle-branch block (RBBB), left ventricular ectopic beats, tricuspid stenosis, atrial septal defect, and Ebstein's anomaly. (See *Auscultating for abnormal S₁ split.*)

Second heart sound

S_2 results from cardiac vibrations caused by closure of the aortic and pulmonic valves as well as the sudden deceleration of blood in the aorta and pulmonary artery. S_2 is usually louder than S_1 at the heart's base and usually slightly higher in pitch than S_1 at the heart's apex. S_2, like S_1, has two basic components:

- the aortic component (A_2)
- the pulmonic component (P_2).

Both of these valves close at the end of ventricular systole. Normally, the aortic valve closes slightly ahead of the pulmonic valve because closing pressure is higher in the aorta than in the pulmonary artery. Therefore, A_2 usually occurs earlier and is louder than P_2. **(SOUND 5)** (See *Valves involved in S₂.*)

Valves involved in S$_2$

When you hear the second heart sound (S$_2$), you're listening to the closing of the aortic and pulmonic valves, shown here.

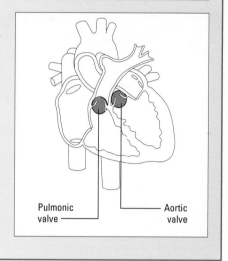

Pulmonic valve

Aortic valve

When the right and left ventricles contract at slightly different times, the sounds are most commonly noted as a split S$_2$. This split isn't abnormal but, occasionally, it can indicate an abnormality such as enlargement of one of the ventricles.

S$_2$ is usually heard best near the base of the heart, over the pulmonic area or over Erb's point. (See *Auscultating for S$_2$, A$_2$, and P$_2$, page 62.*)

Other characteristics of S$_2$ include:

- intensity directly related to the amount of closing pressure in the aorta and pulmonary artery
- slightly shorter duration than S$_1$
- high pitch that's heard best with the diaphragm of the stethoscope
- booming quality
- timing coinciding with the end of ventricular systole. **(SOUND 5)**

Normal S$_2$ split

The normal splitting of S$_2$ into the A$_2$ and P$_2$ components is heard best during inspiration over the pulmonic area. A normal S$_2$ split sounds like "lub/dubdub." Remember, inspiration reduces the intrathoracic pressure in the pulmonary artery. This decrease in pressure causes an increase in venous return to the right side of the heart. This increased

Auscultating for S₂, A₂, and P₂

To hear both components of the second heart sound (S₂), listen carefully with the diaphragm of the stethoscope over the pulmonic area and Erb's point. The aortic component (A₂) is usually louder than the pulmonic component (P₂) over the pulmonic area, located at the left 2nd intercostal space; however, if intense enough, it can be heard over the entire precordium. P₂, which is softer than A₂, is usually heard best over the pulmonic area.

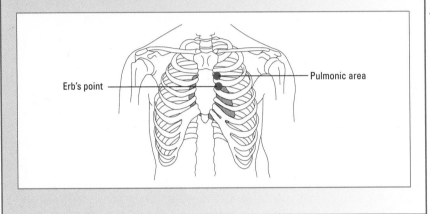

Erb's point

Pulmonic area

venous return delays emptying of the right ventricle, prolonging right ventricular ejection time, and delays closure of the pulmonic valve.

A simultaneous decrease in blood flow to the heart's left side results in a shorter left ventricular ejection time, contributing to the S₂ split. Thus, a normal S₂ split is heard during inspiration. The two sounds normally fuse during expiration. (See *Respiratory changes in normal S₂ split on PCG and ECG.*) **(SOUND 6)**

Changes in A₂ and P₂ intensity

While listening to S₂, you must determine the intensity of the A₂ and P₂ components. Also, note the duration of the A₂–P₂ interval and its relationship to the respiratory cycle. **(SOUND 6)**

You should also document the S₂ split, noting whether the A₂–P₂ interval increases or decreases during inspiration and expiration. The intensity of A₂ and P₂ changes proportionally with the difference in pressure gradients across the closed aortic and pulmonic valves. For

Respiratory changes in normal S₂ split on PCG and ECG

Normal second heart sound (S$_2$) splits are heard best during inspiration. As the patient begins to exhale, the S$_2$ split becomes narrower until it fuses together at expiration. These changes can be seen on this phonocardiogram (PCG) and electrocardiogram (ECG) representation.

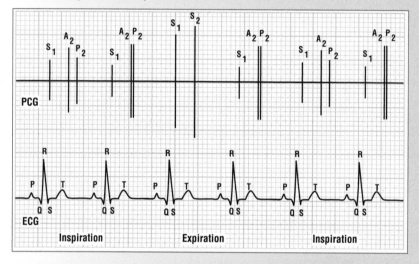

example, P$_2$ may be louder than normal in conditions of elevated pulmonary artery diastolic pressure, as occurs in some patients with heart failure, mitral stenosis, pulmonary hypertension, Eisenmenger's syndrome, or other congenital heart diseases. When P$_2$ increases in intensity, it's sometimes heard over the mitral area and along the left sternal border. **(SOUND 7)**

A$_2$ intensity increases when diastolic pressure in the aorta increases. **(SOUND 8)** This commonly happens:

■ during exercise
■ during states of excitement, including extreme fear
■ in hyperkinetic conditions, such as thyrotoxicosis, fever, and pregnancy
■ in systemic hypertension.

However, if the patient has left ventricular decompensation, ventricular relaxation is slower, and the pressure gradients may not be great enough to produce an accentuated A_2.

Conversely, A_2 intensity may be diminished in conditions that alter the development of diastolic pressure gradients, such as aortic insufficiency and hypotension. **(SOUND 9)** A_2 intensity also decreases when ventricular dysfunction is present, such as after an acute myocardial infarction. In this condition, P_2 may become louder if pulmonary artery pressure rises and systemic pressure falls. A_2 is also softer or absent when aortic valve motion is restricted, as in severe aortic stenosis.

Abnormal S_2 split

Abnormal splitting is related to valvular dysfunction, alterations in blood flow to or from the ventricles, or both. These changes may cause the normal S_2 split to be absent during both phases of the respiratory cycle. Thus, only a single S_2 is heard over Erb's point. In another case, the split sounds may persist through inspiration and expiration with little or no respiratory variation. **(SOUND 10)**

The split sounds may also be heard inconsistently on expiration. The A_2–P_2 intervals vary, as do the intensities of A_2 and P_2 during the respiratory cycle. **(SOUND 11)** Changes in S_2 splits are usually most noticeable at the beginning of inspiration and expiration.

Absent S_2 split

The P_2 component may not be heard during auscultation over Erb's point in a patient with severe pulmonic stenosis. Consequently, S_2 remains a single sound during inspiration and expiration. A normal S_2 split may also be absent if the A_2 sound masks the P_2 sound or vice versa—for example, when one sound is significantly louder than the other, making splitting inaudible. This phenomenon occurs in patients with pulmonary hypertension. In contrast, systemic hypertension causes A_2 to be delayed and to fuse with P_2 during inspiration. In a patient with an increased anteroposterior chest dimension, the P_2 intensity may be so diminished that only A_2 is audible.

Persistent S_2 split

A persistent S_2 split occurs when A_2 and P_2 don't fuse into one sound during expiration. Rather, the split sounds persist throughout inspiration and expiration, even though some respiratory variation in the intensity of A_2 and P_2 is heard. **(SOUND 12)** This persistent A_2–P_2 split-

Persistent S₂ split on PCG and ECG

In a persistent second heart sound (S_2) split, the aortic (A_2) and pulmonic (P_2) components don't fuse during inspiration or expiration. Although the components persist, their intensity may decrease with inspiration and increase with expiration, as shown on this phonocardiogram (PCG) and electrocardiogram (ECG) representation.

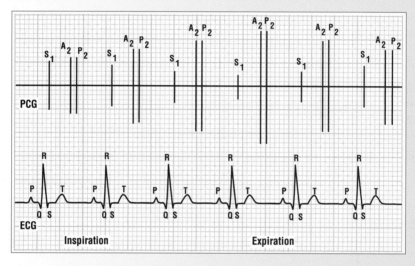

ting during expiration usually results from mitral insufficiency or ventricular septal defect (VSD), which is heard as an early A_2. Atrial septal defect or dilation of the pulmonary artery may be heard as a late P_2. (See *Persistent S_2 split on PCG and ECG*.)

Early aortic valve closure is associated with shortened left ventricular systole, which occurs in patients with mitral insufficiency, VSDs, or cardiac tamponade. Delayed pulmonic valve closure occurs when right ventricular systole is prolonged from structural or physiologic changes or abnormalities, such as in patients with chronic pulmonary hypertension. In these patients, the A_2–P_2 split is heard. The split persists through inspiration and expiration, but the interval between the A_2 and P_2 components is narrowed as compared to the persistent S_2 split. **(SOUND 13)**

Another cause of persistent A_2–P_2 splitting throughout expiration is delayed electrical activation of the right ventricle, which delays P_2.

This phenomenon is commonly found in patients with RBBB, left ventricular epicardial pacing, or left ventricular ectopic beats.

Widened S_2 split

Widened S_2 split may occur during inspiration or expiration. When it occurs during inspiration, it may indicate delayed activation of a contraction or emptying of the right ventricle, resulting in a delayed closing of the pulmonic valve. A widened S_2 split that varies with inspiration is commonly seen in patients with constrictive pericarditis, pulmonic stenosis, or RBBB.

Widened S_2 splits during expiration result from delayed right or left ventricular ejection times. A delayed electrical activation of the right ventricle, resulting in a prolonged right ventricular ejection time, produces expiratory A_2–P_2 splits that are widened and persist even when the patient is seated. **(SOUND 14)** Widened expiratory A_2–P_2 split from prolonged right ventricular ejection time occurs in patients with atrial septal defects, acute or severe pulmonary hypertension secondary to massive pulmonary emboli, or pulmonic stenosis. The P_2 component may not be audible at all in patients with severe pulmonic stenosis. A widened expiratory P_2 split from a delayed left ventricular ejection time may occur in patients with severe mitral insufficiency.

A widened, fixed S_2 split doesn't change with respiration and is associated with the lungs' ability to receive blood volume and the decreased resistance that accompanies that volume. **(SOUND 14)** Wide, fixed splitting occurs when the output of the right ventricle is greater than that of the left ventricle, thus causing a delay in the closing of the pulmonic valve. This phenomenon occurs in patients with idiopathic dilation of the pulmonary artery or large atrial septal defects. A widened, fixed S_2 split may also occur in patients with severe right-sided heart failure when there's little or no increase in right ventricular stroke volume after inspiration or in patients with a VSD with left-to-right shunting. (See *Widened, fixed S_2 split on PCG and ECG.*)

Paradoxical S_2 split

In a paradoxical, or reversed, S_2 split, P_2 precedes A_2, and the split sounds are heard during expiration instead of inspiration.
(SOUND 11) This phenomenon is almost always caused by delayed aortic valve closure. If A_2 is delayed during expiration, it may follow P_2, causing an S_2 split; if A_2 is delayed during inspiration, A_2 and P_2 fuse because inspiration normally delays P_2, causing S_2 to be heard as

Widened, fixed S₂ split on PCG and ECG

Similar to persistent second heart sound (S₂) splits, widened, fixed S₂ splits don't fuse during inspiration or expiration. However, the S₂ split is widened, as shown on this phonocardiogram (PCG) and electrocardiogram (ECG) representation.

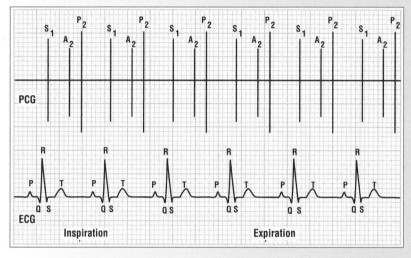

a single sound during inspiration instead of a normally split sound. **(SOUND 15)** (See *Paradoxical S₂ split on PCG and ECG,* page 68.)

KNOW-HOW The mechanics of a paradoxical S₂ split can be remembered this way: Paradox means opposition. So, if A₂ precedes P₂ in a normal S₂ split, then P₂ precedes A₂ in a paradoxical S₂ split. Or, just think about the Ps: in a paradoxical S₂ split, P₂ precedes A₂.

Delayed A₂ is most common in patients with delayed electrical activation of the left ventricle caused by left bundle-branch block (LBBB). LBBB may delay closure of the aortic valve, which normally closes first. This delay causes the pulmonic valve to close first, reversing the usual split and causing P₂–A₂. LBBB is also linked to right ventricular endocardial pacing and premature right ventricular contractions, as in Wolff-Parkinson-White syndrome.

Paradoxical S₂ splits may also be caused by prolonged left ventricular systole, resulting from prolonged left ventricular ejection time. In this case, increased left ventricular stroke volume or increased resist-

Paradoxical S₂ split on PCG and ECG

Unlike normal second heart sound (S₂) splits, paradoxical S₂ splits occur during expiration rather than during inspiration because the aortic component (A₂), rather than the pulmonic component (P₂), is delayed, as shown on this phonocardiogram (PCG) and electrocardiogram (ECG) representation. During inspiration, the components fuse together into one sound, S₂.

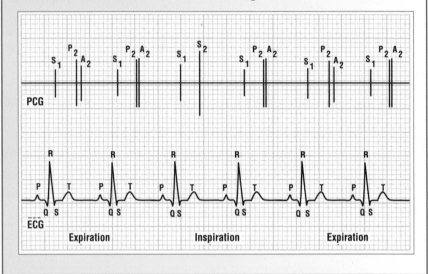

ance to left ventricular ejection may cause left ventricular pressure overload.

Left ventricular overload from increased left ventricular stroke volume is commonly seen in aortic insufficiency and patent ductus arteriosus. However, the paradoxical split is rarely heard. Left ventricular overload, usually because of left-sided heart failure, commonly occurs in patients with systemic hypertension and hypertrophic cardiomyopathy. Aortic stenosis may also lead to paradoxical splitting of A₂ and P₂; however, if stenosis is severe, the A₂ component may not be audible.

6 S_3 and S_4 heart sounds

The first and second heart sounds, S_1 and S_2, mark the beginning and end, respectively, of ventricular systole and associated valve closures. In healthy people, these two sounds and their components are relatively easy to hear during auscultation and are best heard with the diaphragm of the stethoscope.

The two left ventricular diastolic filling sounds, S_3 and S_4, are sometimes heard over the mitral area. These sounds differ from S_1 and S_2 in that they're low-frequency sounds and are produced by ventricular filling rather than by valve closures.

Third heart sound

Occasionally, a physiologic S_3 is heard during auscultation after S_2. S_3 sounds are caused by vibrations occurring during rapid, passive ventricular filling. Early in diastole, after isovolumic relaxation, the mitral and tricuspid valves open, and the ventricles fill and expand. (See *Understanding S_3*, page 70.)

S_3 is normal in children, healthy people younger than age 20, and very athletic young adults. In children and young adults, the left ventricle is normally compliant, permitting rapid filling. The left ventricle responds with an abrupt change in wall motion that causes a sudden decrease in blood flow. These events generate vibrations, which are responsible for physiologic S_3. The more vigorously the left ventricle expands, the greater the chance that an S_3 will occur.

A physiologic S_3 is also commonly audible in patients with high-output conditions, in which rapid ventricular expansion is caused by increased blood volume. Anemia, fever, pregnancy, and thyrotoxicosis

Understanding S₃

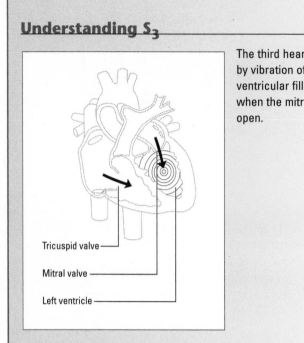

The third heart sound (S₃) is caused by vibration of the ventricles during ventricular filling, which occurs when the mitral and tricuspid valves open.

Tricuspid valve

Mitral valve

Left ventricle

are some of the conditions that cause rapid ventricular expansion, resulting in an S_3.

An S_3 is also commonly heard in:

- young, slender people during periods of excessive catecholamine release such as in pheochromocytoma
- acute myocardial infarction (MI)
- acute alcohol withdrawal
- cocaine abuse
- stroke
- severe heart failure.

In older adults and elderly patients, an S_3 may be the first indication of heart failure.

Auscultating for S₃

To listen for a third heart sound (S₃), place your stethoscope over the mitral area, located in the 5th intercostal space at the midclavicular line (shown below).

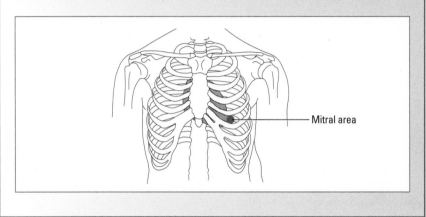

Mitral area

Characteristics of S₃

S₃ is usually heard best near the apex of the heart, over the mitral area. (See *Auscultating for S₃*.)

Characteristics include:

■ varying intensity and loudness (sometimes soft, faint, and difficult to hear and other times loud and easy to hear)

■ best heard during expiration when blood flow into the left ventricle is increased **(SOUND 16)**

■ short duration

■ possibly intermittent occurrence with every third or fourth heartbeat

■ dull, thudlike quality.

S₃ is heard early in diastole. Its timing is closely related to S₂, which is heard just after the T wave, and follows S₂ by 0.14 to 0.20 second. **(SOUND 16)** The relationship of S₃ to the electrocardiogram (ECG) waveform can be seen easily on a phonocardiogram (PCG); on the ECG, S₃ occurs during the TP interval just after the T wave. Normally, the S₂-S₃ interval is reliably constant. (See *Physiologic S₃ on PCG and ECG*, page 72.)

Physiologic S₃ on PCG and ECG

A third heart sound (S₃) usually follows a second heart sound (S₂) by 0.14 to 0.20 second. The timing is relatively constant between the TP intervals, as shown on this phonocardiogram (PCG) and electrocardiogram (ECG) representation.

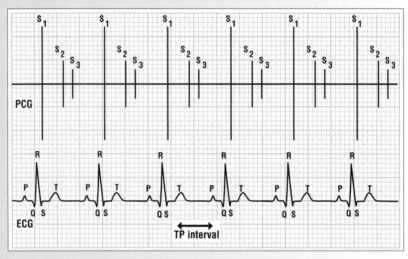

KNOW-HOW *Here are some tips to enhance your ability to auscultate and palpate S₃:*

■ *Place the patient in a partial left lateral recumbent position.*

■ *Usually, S₃ is heard best with the bell of the stethoscope over the mitral area, and it can usually be palpated over the same area.*

■ *Because S₃ is associated with blood volume and velocity, it can be intensified by maneuvers that increase stroke volume, such as elevating the patient's legs from a recumbent position or having the patient exercise briefly or cough several times.*

■ *S₃ commonly disappears with maneuvers that decrease venous return, such as having the patient sit up or stand.*

Abnormal S₃

As a person ages, the heart's left ventricle becomes less compliant. Decreased ventricular compliance leads to pressure changes, which cause

Understanding abnormal S₃

An abnormal third heart sound (S_3) occurs when the left ventricle becomes less compliant or thickened, which may occur with increased age.

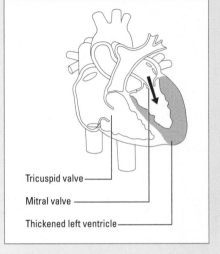

Tricuspid valve

Mitral valve

Thickened left ventricle

slowed left ventricular isovolumic relaxation and reduced blood flow velocity into the ventricle. (See *Understanding abnormal S_3*.)

Gallop

An audible S_3 in a person older than age 20 is abnormal unless the person is a highly trained athlete. This abnormal S_1-S_2-S_3 sequence is referred to as a ventricular gallop or gallop rhythm. **(SOUND 17)** An abnormal S_3 has the same sound characteristics, is heard over the same location (the mitral area), and has the same timing in relation to S_2 as a physiologic S_3. The differences between the two are related to the patient's age and clinical condition. Also, an S_3 gallop rhythm usually persists despite maneuvers that decrease venous return. **(SOUND 17)**

An abnormal S_3 is heard in conditions of increased blood volume and increased inflow velocity into the left ventricle. Ventricular diastolic pressure may or may not be increased. Consequently, a patient with mitral insufficiency or heart failure may have an abnormal S_3. This heart sound can also be heard during increased blood flow through the mitral valve, which occurs in patients with ventricular septal defects, patent ductus arteriosus, or severe aortic insufficiency. (See *Responding to heart failure,* page 74.)

CASE CLIP

Responding to heart failure

Mrs. S. is an 84-year-old female well-known to her practitioner for a history of cardiomyopathy with an ejection fraction at 20%. She has had recurrent problems with exacerbations of heart failure. She presented to the office stating, "I'm in heart failure again." She complained of increased shortness of breath (SOB), increased lower extremity edema, nocturnal dyspnea to the point she had slept in her recliner the past 2 evenings because she couldn't breathe comfortably laying in bed. She was admitted to the hospital for I.V. diuresis, inotropic support, and medication adjustment.

Initially, Mrs. S. responded well to treatment, her edema and dyspnea resolved over 2 days. Her practitioner discussed with her that he wanted to continue I.V. medication therapy and electrocardiogram monitoring for 1 more day. Throughout the rest of the day, Mrs. S. noticed she was experiencing a return of her SOB. Mrs. S. didn't notify the nurse of the changes until she was extremely short of breath even at rest. The evening nurse noted on her initial assessment that Mrs. S. was in respiratory distress with labored respirations. Vital signs at this time were:
- temperature: 97.6° F (36.4° C)
- heart rate: 98 beats/minute
- respiratory rate: 36 breaths/minute
- blood pressure: 72/36 mm Hg
- pulse oximetry: 78% on room air.

Breath sounds revealed bibasilar crackles and scattered wheezes, jugular vein distention was present, 1+ pitting edema. On auscultation, there was an S_1, S_2, and S_3 gallop.

Realizing Mrs. S. was in distress the rapid response team (RRT) was called. While waiting for the RRT to respond, the nurse assisted Mrs. S. into a comfortable position with the head of bed elevated, and placed her on oxygen at 6 L/minute via nasal cannula. Staff from the floor responded quickly to the call for assistance and, prior to the RRT's arrival, had Mrs. S. on a defibrillator/monitor with continuous pulse oximetry reading. Mrs. S. was assessed by the RRT and based on her deteriorating condition was diagnosed with pulmonary edema. The RRT intubated Mrs. S. for respiratory support and treated her with additional furosemide and bronchodilators. Mrs. S.'s practitioner was notified and informed of the transfer to intensive care unit (ICU). A chest X-ray, done to confirm endotracheal tube placement, revealed findings consistent with heart failure. Samples were sent to the laboratory on admission to the ICU and an elevated brain natriuretic peptide serum level of 1,500 pg/ml—with the normal range being 0 to 100 pg/ml—was reported.

Treatment for Mrs. S.'s heart failure included I.V. diuretics and a continuous infusion of an inotropic medication for 24 hours. Mrs. S. was extubated the next day and spent 7 inpatient days recovering and was discharged home in fair condition on an angiotensin-converting inhibitor and an angiotensin II receptor blocker.

Auscultating for pericardial knock

Pericardial knock is heard best over the 3rd, 4th, and 5th intercostal spaces along the left sternal border, as shown here.

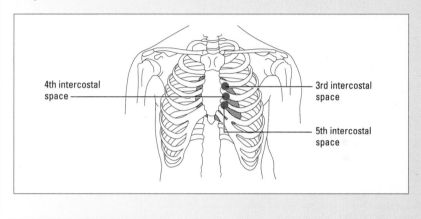

4th intercostal space

3rd intercostal space

5th intercostal space

Pericardial knock

An abnormal S_3 in patients with constrictive pericarditis is called *pericardial knock.* This type of abnormal S_3 occurs closer to S_2. The interval between S_2 and S_3 is usually less than 0.14 second. **(SOUND 18)** With the diaphragm of the stethoscope, the pericardial knock is easier to hear than a normal or abnormal S_3. **(SOUND 18)** Inspiration usually intensifies pericardial knock. (See *Auscultating for pericardial knock.*)

Right-sided S_3

Because the right ventricle is normally much more compliant than the left ventricle, its filling shouldn't cause vibrations that create an S_3. However, in some patients, an S_3 originates in the right ventricle instead of the left. When it does, it's always an abnormality. **(SOUND 19)** Right-sided S_3 is more prominent during inspiration because of increased blood flow into the right ventricle. (See *Understanding right-sided S_3,* page 76.)

Patients with enlarged right ventricles commonly have right-sided S_3. This heart sound is audible in patients with right-sided heart failure, pulmonic insufficiency, or severe tricuspid insufficiency. **(SOUND 19)** (See *Auscultating for right-sided S_3,* page 76.)

Understanding right-sided S₃

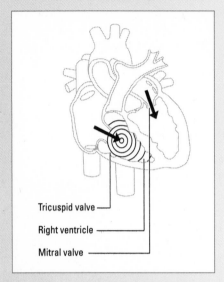

It's easy to remember that a right-sided third heart sound (S₃) occurs when the right ventricle isn't compliant. Right-sided S₃ is abnormal.

Tricuspid valve

Right ventricle

Mitral valve

Auscultating for right-sided S₃

A right-sided third heart sound (S₃) is heard best over the 3rd, 4th, and 5th intercostal spaces and over the epigastric area.

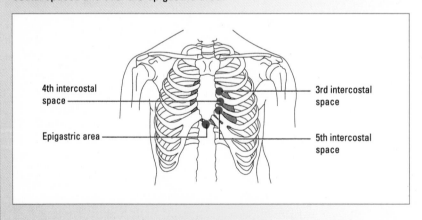

4th intercostal space

3rd intercostal space

Epigastric area

5th intercostal space

Fourth heart sound

By the end of diastole, the ventricles are nearly full; atrial contraction further stretches and fills them. The vibrations caused by this stretching and filling in late diastole generate an additional heart sound, S_4, sometimes called an *atrial diastolic gallop*. **(SOUND 20)** (See *Understanding S_4.*)

An S_4 is almost always abnormal, except in highly trained young athletes with physiologic left ventricular hypertrophy. Because S_4 is linked to atrial contraction, it isn't produced in conditions in which atrial systole doesn't occur, such as atrial fibrillation.

Characteristics of S_4

Usually, S_4 is located near the heart's apex over the mitral area; occasionally, it's also palpable over this area. (See *Auscultating for S_4*, page 78.)

Other characteristics of S_4 include:
- varying intensity and loudness (sometimes faint and difficult to hear; other times, loud and easy to hear)

Understanding S_4

A fourth heart sound (S_4) is produced when the ventricles are filling and stretching.

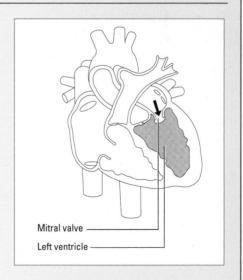

Mitral valve ——————

Left ventricle ——————

Auscultating for S₄

To best hear a fourth heart sound (S₄), place the bell of the stethoscope over the mitral area, as shown here.

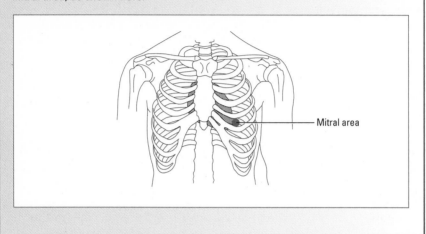

Mitral area

- relatively short duration and intermittent occurrence with every third or fourth heartbeat
- low pitch that's best heard with the bell of the stethoscope
- thudlike quality
- presystolic timing
- relationship to S₁ that's easily seen in the ECG waveform
- occurrence during PR interval and before S₁. **(SOUND 20)** (See *S₄ on PCG and ECG.*)

Abnormal S₄

An abnormal S₄ almost always occurs with increased mean left atrial pressure caused by a noncompliant left ventricle. It's heard during or after an acute MI as well as in patients with:

- hypertension (the most common cause)
- cardiomyopathies, especially hypertrophic cardiomyopathy
- ischemic heart disease.

When S₄ occurs in a patient with hypertension, systolic blood pressure usually exceeds 160 mm Hg or diastolic pressure exceeds 100 mm Hg.

S₄ on PCG and ECG

A fourth heart sound (S_4) is easy to see on the phonocardiogram (PCG) and electrocardiogram (ECG) representation below. S_4 occurs before the first heart sound (S_1) during the PR interval.

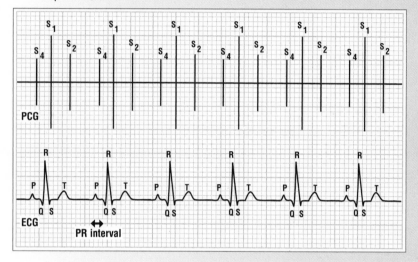

An abnormal S_4 can also accompany certain volume overload conditions, such as:

- hyperthyroidism
- certain anemias
- sudden severe mitral insufficiency.

Summation gallop

Normally, S_4 precedes S_1 by an appreciable interval that correlates with the PR interval on the ECG. However, in patients with first-degree atrioventricular block, the P wave occurs early in diastole, and S_4 may occur during the early rapid diastolic filling period.

Likewise, in tachycardia, S_4 may cover up S_3 during early rapid filling. If either of these conditions exists, the S_4 fuses with S_3 to become a single diastolic filling sound called a *summation gallop,* which may be louder than S_4, S_3, or S_1. **(SOUND 21)** (See *Summation gallop on PCG and ECG,* page 80.)

Summation gallop on PCG and ECG

In summation gallop, a fourth heart sound (S₄) may occur early or cover up the third heart sound (S₃), thus becoming a single diastolic filling sound. Summation gallop may be louder than S₄, S₃, and the first heart sound (S₁). The pattern is shown on this phonocardiogram (PCG) and electrocardiogram (ECG) representation.

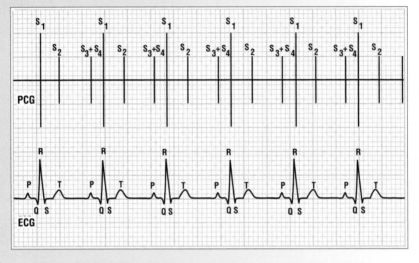

Understanding right-sided S₄

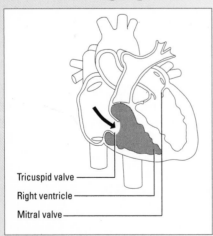

A right-sided fourth heart sound (S₄) appears when S₄ occurs in the right ventricle instead of the left, as shown here.

Tricuspid valve

Right ventricle

Mitral valve

Auscultating for right-sided S₄

A right-sided fourth heart sound (S₄) is heard best over the 3rd, 4th, and 5th intercostal spaces along the left sternal border and over the epigastric area (shown here) with the patient in a supine position.

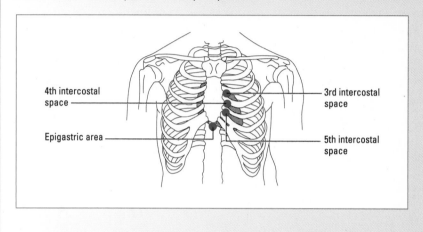

4th intercostal space

Epigastric area

3rd intercostal space

5th intercostal space

Right-sided S₄

S₄ generated in the right ventricle is called a right-sided S₄. **(SOUND 22)** (See *Understanding right-sided S₄*.) It's commonly heard in conditions that increase pressure in the right ventricle by more than 100 mm Hg, such as pulmonic stenosis or pulmonary hypertension. Although the sound may vary with respiration, it's more audible during inspiration. (See *Auscultating for right-sided S₄*.)

Differentiating S₄ from S₁ split

Distinguishing an S₁ split (M₁–T₁) from an S₄–S₁ sequence is sometimes difficult. Here are some tips to help you distinguish them:
■ An S₁ split is best heard between the mitral and tricuspid areas with the diaphragm of the stethoscope, whereas an S₄ is best heard over the mitral area with the bell of the stethoscope and usually isn't audible with the diaphragm.
■ An S₄ may be palpable.
■ An S₁ split is a systolic ejection sound, which is higher in pitch than S₄.

S_3 and S_4: Similarities and differences

S_3, like S_4, is low-pitched and may be faint or loud and heard only intermittently. Both sounds are heard best at the heart's apex, located over the mitral area, using the bell of the stethoscope, with the patient in a partial left lateral recumbent position. Both sounds vary with respirations and can be enhanced by maneuvers that increase stroke volume, such as elevating the patient's legs while in a recumbent position or having him perform handgrip exercises.

At times, differentiating S_3 from S_4 is difficult. Remember that S_3 is heard after S_2, whereas S_4 occurs at the beginning of atrial systole and therefore occurs before S_1.

7 *Other diastolic and systolic sounds*

In previous chapters, you've learned about several types of heart sounds, including S_1, S_2, S_3, and S_4. This chapter reviews other systolic and diastolic sounds, including opening snap, systolic ejection sound, pulmonic ejection sound, aortic ejection sound, and midsystolic click.

Opening snap

At the end of ventricular systole, the aortic and pulmonic valves close, generating the second heart sound (S_2). S_2 is followed by a brief period of isovolumic relaxation; during this time, ventricular pressure falls. When ventricular pressure is less than atrial pressure, the mitral and tricuspid valves open. In a healthy heart, the mitral and tricuspid valves open silently during diastole. In certain pathologic states, these atrioventricular valves will open more rapidly than normal and make a sound known as an *opening snap* (OS). This snapping sound occurs when valve leaflets become stenotic or abnormally narrowed (as in patients with a history of rheumatic fever) while remaining somewhat mobile. **(SOUND 23)** (See *Understanding an OS,* page 84.)

Causes of mitral valve OS include:

- mitral stenosis (most common)
- mitral stenosis with a mobile valve
- rapid mitral flow, which causes a soft snap (such as left-to-right shunt in ventricular septal defect or patent ductus arteriosus)
- severe mitral insufficiency.

A tricuspid OS is rare but may be caused by:

Understanding an OS

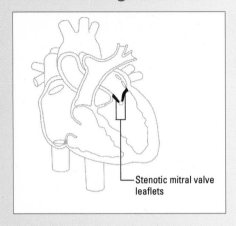

An opening snap (OS) is caused by stenotic but mobile mitral valve leaflets. The location of these leaflets is shown here.

Stenotic mitral valve leaflets

- tricuspid valve abnormalities (as in rheumatic stenosis)
- increased tricuspid flow (as in left-to-right shunt in an atrial septal defect).

An OS is generated by maximum opening of the leaflets, which is somewhat limited because of stenosis. The OS usually marks the beginning of a diastolic murmur in mitral stenosis. The intensity of the OS is directly proportional to the motility of the valve and the degree of fusion of the valve's cusps. The timing of the OS is influenced by atrial pressure (higher pressure equals earlier snap) and the duration of the isovolumetric relaxation phase (shorter relaxation phase equals earlier OS). If the mitral valve becomes severely calcified and inflexible, the OS disappears.

Characteristics of an OS

An OS is usually heard best near the heart's apex over the mitral area or just medial to it. (See *Auscultating for an OS*.) Intensity varies among patients; however, it's usually easy to hear during auscultation. To distinguish the OS from P_2, auscultate heart sounds during inspiration to hear A_2, P_2, and the OS in quick succession.

Other sound characteristics include:
- short duration
- high pitch that's heard best with the diaphragm of the stethoscope

Auscultating for an OS

An opening snap (OS) is heard best with the diaphragm of the stethoscope near the heart's apex over the mitral area (shown here) or just medial to it. An OS is also transmitted widely across the precordium and usually can be heard over the aortic, pulmonic, and tricuspid areas.

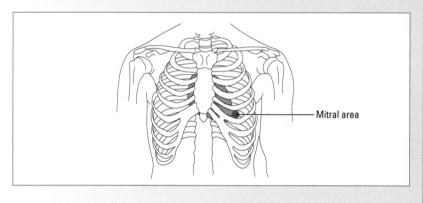

Mitral area

- distinctive sharp, crisp, snaplike quality
- higher pitch than S_2
- as loud as or louder than S_2
- timing closely related to S_2
- occurrence early in ventricular diastole, just after the stenotic mitral valve opens
- occurrence just after the T wave in the electrocardiogram (ECG) waveform. **(SOUND 23)** (See *OS on PCG and ECG,* page 86.)

Differentiating OS from S₂

An OS occurs early in diastole and may be confused with the pulmonic component (P_2) or the third heart sound (S_3). One characteristic of an OS that helps distinguish it from P_2 is its timing: The aortic component (A_2)–P_2 interval is normally shorter than the A_2–OS interval. Also, when the patient stands, the A_2–P_2 interval narrows, whereas the A_2–OS interval widens.

Another characteristic is that the A_2–OS interval remains constant throughout respiration, whereas the A_2–P_2 interval normally widens during inspiration and narrows during expiration. During inspiration,

OS on PCG and ECG

An opening snap (OS) arises soon after the second heart sound (S_2), just after the T wave, as shown on this phonocardiogram (PCG) and electrocardiogram (ECG) representation.

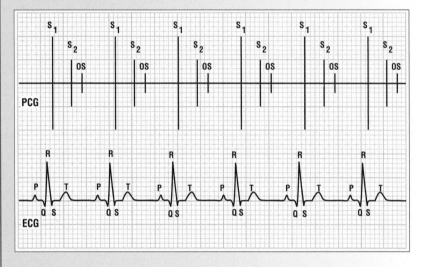

three distinct sounds can usually be heard over the pulmonic area; therefore, the sequence must be A_2, P_2, OS. In contrast, during expiration, the A_2–P_2 interval narrows or fuses, forming one sound. This creates an S_2–OS interval.

Finally, P_2 isn't usually heard over the mitral area. Therefore, if you hear a split S_2 over this area, it may be an S_2 and an OS.

Differentiating OS from S_3

Distinguishing an OS from an S_3 is difficult in some patients, especially those with mild mitral stenosis when the A_2–OS interval is wider than usual and the OS is somewhat softer. One characteristic of an OS that helps distinguish it from an S_3 is its timing. Also, the A_2–S_3 interval is usually longer than the A_2–OS interval. Furthermore, S_3 is a low-frequency sound that's heard best over the mitral area with the bell of the stethoscope. In contrast, an OS produces a high-frequency

KNOW-HOW

Tips for hearing an OS

When auscultating for an opening snap (OS) of the mitral valve, remember that it has a quality similar to a normal heart sound and is commonly confused with a split S_2. The brief, sharp, snapping sound is heard shortly after the aortic component (A_2) of S_2.

Stethoscope for snap
To hear an OS better, place the stethoscope midway between the pulmonic and mitral areas. A loud OS will be widely transmitted over the entire precordium. In addition, turn the patient to the left lateral position because standing tends to lower left atrial pressure and thus increase the A_2–OS interval.

Exercise intensifies
Remember that a soft OS may be intensified after exercise, which increases atrial pressure. Although the A_2–OS interval isn't altered during different phases of respiration, a mitral valve OS is usually heard loudest on expiration.

---

sound that's more widely transmitted across the precordium and is heard best with the diaphragm.

Another characteristic of an OS is that its intensity usually isn't affected by having the patient stand, whereas S_3 intensity can be increased by increasing stroke volume through such activities as standing, coughing, or exercising briefly. Finally, if the murmur typically heard in patients with mitral stenosis is present, you can confirm that the sound is an OS. (See *Tips for hearing an OS*.)

Systolic ejection sound

Just as an OS is caused by stenotic mitral valve leaflets, a systolic ejection sound (SES) is caused by the opening of a stenotic aortic or pulmonic valve. Systolic ejection murmurs are discussed in depth in chapter 9; however, here's a short overview on SESs.

An SES usually occurs early in systole after S_1 and isovolumic contraction. It's commonly associated with ventricular ejection and the maximum opening of a stenotic, yet mobile, aortic or pulmonic valve.

Understanding an SES

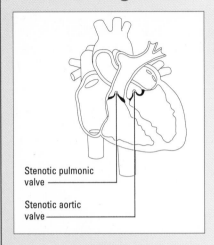

A systolic ejection sound (SES) arises from a stenotic but mobile aortic or pulmonic valve. The locations of these valves are shown here.

Stenotic pulmonic valve

Stenotic aortic valve

If the valve is severely stenotic because of calcification, an SES—like an OS—won't occur. (See *Understanding an SES.*)

It also may be caused by sudden distention of an already dilated aorta or pulmonary artery and by forceful ventricular ejection from pulmonary or systemic hypertension. An SES is abnormal whether it originates in the heart's right or left side.

Pulmonic ejection sound

A pulmonic ejection sound (PES) is the only right-sided heart sound that increases in intensity during expiration and diminishes or disappears during inspiration. **(SOUND 24)**

In a normal heart, inspiration increases right ventricular volume, causing the pulmonic leaflet valve to form a dome shape toward the pulmonary artery, which decreases the sound's intensity. During expiration, right ventricular volume is decreased, the valve leaflet is less domed, and its opening produces a louder snap. In a patient with pulmonary artery dilation or pulmonary hypertension, a PES may not vary in intensity during respiration.

Auscultating for a PES

You can best hear a pulmonic ejection sound (PES) when you place your stethoscope over the pulmonic area (shown here).

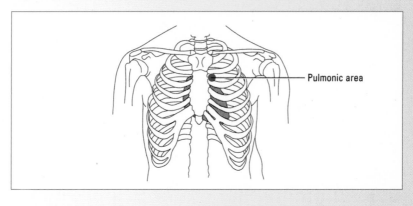

Pulmonic area

Because a PES may occur in idiopathic dilation of the pulmonary artery but usually isn't present in supravalvular or muscular subvalvular obstructions, its presence can be used to differentiate these conditions. Occasionally, a PES may also be heard with atrial and ventricular septal defects.

Characteristics of a PES

A PES usually is heard best near the heart's base over the pulmonic area. (See *Auscultating for a PES.*)

Other sound characteristics include:

- soft intensity (may be equal to or greater than that of S_1)
- short duration
- a high pitch that's heard best with the diaphragm of the stethoscope
- a sharp or clicklike quality
- timing that's closely related to the first heart sound (S_1)
- occurrence early in ventricular systole, just after the opening of a stenotic pulmonic valve **(SOUND 24)**
- occurrence just after the QRS complex. (See *PES on PCG and ECG,* page 90.)

PES on PCG and ECG

A pulmonic ejection sound (PES) is closely related to the first heart sound (S₁). It occurs just after S₁, after the QRS complex, as shown on this phonocardiogram (PCG) and electrocardiogram (ECG) representation.

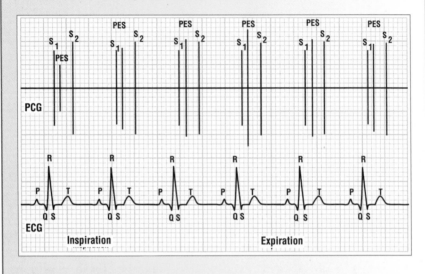

To differentiate a pulmonic ejection sound (PES) from an S₁, remember that a PES is heard in the pulmonic area and varies with respiration. A split S₁ is heard in the tricuspid area and doesn't vary with respiration.

Aortic ejection sound

Unlike a PES, which is caused by pulmonic valve stenosis, an aortic ejection sound (AES) is caused by aortic valve stenosis. This sound doesn't vary in intensity with respiration.

An AES may occur in patients with aortic root dilation, which is commonly associated with such conditions as systemic hypertension, an ascending aortic aneurysm, or coarctation of the aorta. An AES may also be heard in patients with aortic stenosis or aortic insufficiency, but the sound is less clicklike when it's associated with aortic insufficiency. **(SOUND 25)**

Auscultating for an AES

An aortic ejection sound (AES) has a high pitch. To listen for an AES, place your stethoscope over any of the areas shown here.

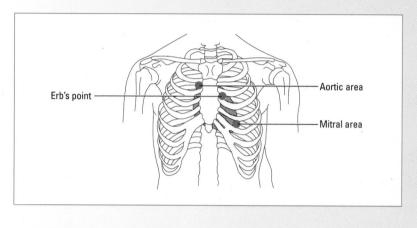

Erb's point

Aortic area

Mitral area

Characteristics of an AES

An AES is heard best near the heart's apex over the mitral area, near the heart's base over the aortic area, or over Erb's point. (See *Auscultating for an AES.*)

Other sound characteristics include:

- soft intensity (may be equal to or greater than that of S_1)
- short duration
- high pitch that's heard best with the diaphragm of the stethoscope
- sharp or clicklike quality
- timing that's closely related to S_1 **(SOUND 25)**
- occurrence early in ventricular systole, just after the opening of a stenotic aortic valve
- occurrence just after the QRS complex in the ECG waveform.

Certain characteristics help to distinguish an AES from other heart sounds. One such characteristic is that an AES radiates more than a PES. Another characteristic is that a split S_1 heard over the mitral area is more likely to be a mitral component than an AES.

You can differentiate an AES from a fourth heart sound (S_4) by remembering that S_4 is heard best with the bell of the stethoscope over the mitral area and is usually accompanied by a palpable, presystolic apical bulge. Also, an S_4 is intensified by maneuvers that increase left atrial pressure, such as brief exercise, squatting, or coughing. An AES isn't affected by any of these maneuvers.

Midsystolic click

A midsystolic click (MSC) occurs when the prolapsed mitral valve's leaflets and chordae tendineae become tense. The anterior or posterior leaflet, or both leaflets, can prolapse. Occasionally, multiple clicks occur that are heard in midsystole to late systole; they're heard best over the tricuspid area and toward the mitral area. Like an ejection sound, these midsystolic to late-systolic clicks are crisp, high-frequency sounds. **(SOUND 26)** (See *Understanding an MSC.*)

Characteristics of an MSC

An MSC usually is heard best over the tricuspid area and near the heart's apex over the mitral area. (See *Auscultating for an MSC.*)

Other characteristics include:
- intensity equal to or greater than that of S_1
- short duration
- high pitch that's heard best with the diaphragm of the stethoscope

Understanding an MSC

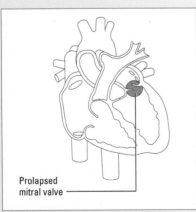

Prolapsed
mitral valve

Midsystolic click (MSC) occurs when the anterior or posterior mitral valve leaflets prolapse and the chordae tendineae tense, as shown here.

Auscultating for an MSC

To best hear a midsystolic click (MSC), place your stethoscope over the tricuspid and mitral areas (shown here).

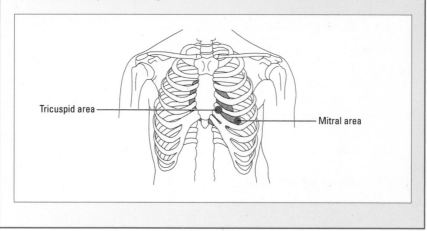

Tricuspid area

Mitral area

- clicklike quality
- variability of the click's timing, occurring in early systole, midsystole, or late systole
- occurrence during QT interval on the ECG waveform. **(SOUND 26)** (See *MSC on PCG and ECG,* page 94.)

The timing of an MSC is affected by certain movements, such as having the patient stand or performing Valsalva's maneuver. Such maneuvers reduce left ventricular filling and cause the MSC to be heard closer to S_1. The MSC may even merge with S_1 or disappear completely. Increasing left ventricular volume by raising the legs from a recumbent position or squatting delays the click. This maneuver may also cause the prolapse not to occur and the MSC to be diminished or inaudible.

Sometimes an MSC is accompanied by a late systolic crescendo murmur or the characteristic holosystolic murmur of mitral insufficiency. An MSC may also be caused by such extracardiac conditions as pleuropericardial adhesions, atrial septal aneurysms, and cardiac tumors.

MSC on PCG and ECG

A midsystolic click (MSC) occurs during the QT interval, as shown on this phono-cardiogram (PCG) and electrocardiogram (ECG) representation.

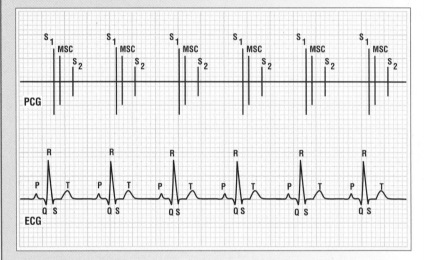

8 Murmur fundamentals

Murmurs

A murmur is an abnormal, usually periodic sound of short duration that's heard during auscultation. A murmur may be benign or may be caused by a medical condition. Many different types of murmurs exist; specific murmur types are discussed in later chapters.

Causes

Whereas heart sounds are produced by brief vibrations that correspond to the beginning and end of systole, murmurs are produced by a prolonged series of vibrations that occur during systole and diastole. These vibrations result from turbulent blood flow.

Longer than a heart sound, a murmur occurs as a vibrating, blowing, or rumbling noise. Just as water in a stream "babbles" as it passes through a narrow point, turbulent blood flow produces a murmur.

Several conditions—such as blood flowing at a high velocity through a partially obstructed opening, blood flowing from a higher pressure chamber to a lower pressure one, or any combination of these—can cause turbulent blood flow. Other causes of turbulence include structural defects in the heart's chambers or valves and changes in the viscosity of the blood or the speed of blood flow. You may hear these heart murmurs over the same precordial areas during auscultation. (See *Tips for listening to murmurs,* page 96, and *Differentiating murmurs,* pages 97 and 98.)

KNOW-HOW

Tips for listening to murmurs

Here are some tips that can help improve your murmur auscultation:

■ Initially, learn to identify the loudest location and pinpoint the timing of murmurs.

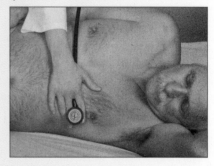

■ As your auscultation techniques improve, try to identify the intensity, duration, pitch, quality, and configuration.

■ The best way to hear murmurs is with the patient sitting up and leaning forward. You can also ask the patient to lie on his left side, as shown here.

Murmur characteristics

Like other heart sounds, murmurs are described by several characteristics heard during auscultation. The terms used to describe a specific characteristic are determined mainly by the volume and speed of blood flow as blood moves through the heart.

Make sure to describe murmurs carefully and accurately so you can easily recognize changes in a patient's murmur characteristics and immediately assess the possible source of those changes. Seven characteristics are used to describe murmurs:

■ location
■ intensity
■ duration
■ pitch
■ quality
■ timing
■ configuration.

Location

A murmur's location is the anatomic area on the chest wall where you can hear it best. This is usually also the murmur's point of maximum intensity. This area typically correlates with the underlying location of the valve that's responsible for producing the murmur. For example, a murmur of aortic stenosis is usually heard best near the heart's base

Differentiating murmurs

SOUND	LOCATION	CAUSE
■ Medium pitch ■ Harsh quality ■ Possibly musical at apex ■ Loudest with expiration ■ Grade 4 or higher	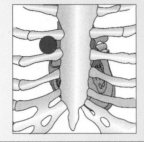	Aortic stenosis
■ Medium pitch ■ Harsh quality ■ Variable-grade intensity	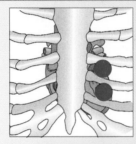	Hypertrophic cardiomyopathy
■ High pitch ■ Blowing quality ■ Grade 1 to 3 intensity	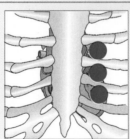	Aortic insufficiency
■ Medium to high pitch ■ Blowing quality ■ Soft to loud grade intensity	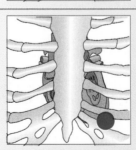	Mitral insufficiency

(continued)

 = Diaphragm    = Bell

Differentiating murmurs *(continued)*

SOUND	LOCATION	CAUSE
▪ Medium to high pitch ▪ Blowing quality ▪ Variable intensity ▪ Increases slightly with inspiration		Tricuspid insufficiency
▪ High pitch ▪ Harsh quality ▪ Grade 5 or 6 intensity		Ventricular septal defect
▪ Low pitch ▪ Rumbling quality ▪ Grade 1 to 4 intensity		Mitral stenosis

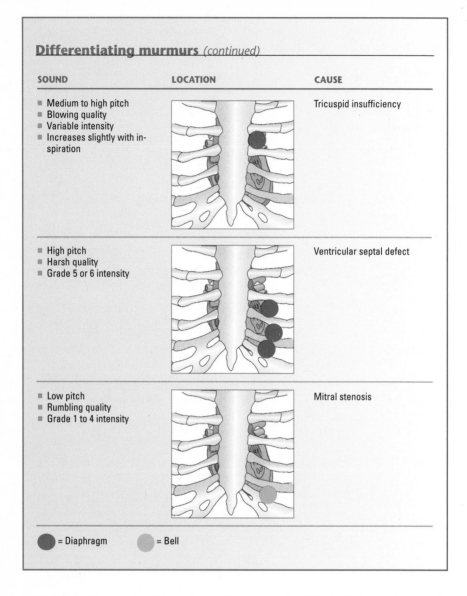

● = Diaphragm   ● = Bell

over the aortic area, whereas a murmur of mitral insufficiency is usually heard best near the heart's apex over the mitral area.

The murmur's sounds also may be transmitted to the chamber or vessel where the turbulent blood flow occurs. This phenomenon, known as *radiation,* occurs because the direction of blood flow determines sound transmission. Murmurs radiate in either a forward or a backward direction (to the neck or axillae).

Intensity

The second characteristic, intensity, refers to the murmur's loudness. Intensity is influenced by a patient's body weight and certain other conditions. For example, because heart sounds are affected by chest wall thickness and by certain diseases, heart sounds and murmurs are usually louder in thin people and fainter in obese people. They're also fainter in patients with emphysema, an abnormal swelling of lung tissue caused by accumulation of air, usually from the loss of elasticity or from alveolar injury.

Hyperdynamic states, decreased blood viscosity, increased pressure gradients across valves, increased blood flow, and faster heart rates also may increase a murmur's intensity. Murmurs are less intense in hypodynamic states and in patients with an elevated hematocrit.

Document a murmur's intensity using a uniform method. Most health care professionals use a six-point graded scale known as the *Levine grading scale,* with I being the faintest intensity and VI being the loudest. (See *Grading murmurs,* page 100.)

Duration

Duration is the length of time you can hear the murmur during systole or diastole. It can be described as long or short.

Pitch

A murmur's pitch, or frequency, can vary from high to medium to low. It's usually higher in conditions of increased blood flow velocity or increased pressure gradients and lower in conditions with lower blood flow velocity.

Quality

A murmur's quality is determined by the combination of frequencies that produces the sound. Words to describe quality may include "harsh," "rough," "musical," "scratchy," "squeaky," "rumbling," or "blowing."

Timing

A murmur's timing refers to when the murmur occurs in the cardiac cycle. This means that you describe the onset, duration, and end of the murmur in relation to systole and diastole. The beginning of systole, or

Grading murmurs

Use the Levine grading scale outlined below to describe a murmur's intensity:
- Grade I murmur is faint, may be heard intermittently, and is barely heard through the stethoscope.
- Grade II murmur is audible but quiet and soft; it's usually heard as soon as the stethoscope is placed on the chest wall.
- Grade III murmur is easily heard and is described as moderately loud.
- Grade IV murmur is loud and usually associated with a palpable vibration known as a *thrill* or *thrust*. It also may radiate in the direction of blood flow.
- Grade V murmur is loud enough to be heard with only an edge of the stethoscope touching the chest wall; it's almost always accompanied by a palpable thrill and radiation.
- Grade VI murmur is so loud that it can be heard with the stethoscope close to, but not touching, the chest wall; it's always accompanied by a palpable thrill, and it radiates to distant structures.

Documenting murmurs

When you document a murmur's grade, use Roman numerals as part of a fraction with VI always listed as the denominator—for example, III/VI. This means you consider the murmur to be a grade III and have used the six-point scale for assessment. That way, all health care professionals will understand which scale you used, even if they don't use the same one.

S_1, can be identified easily by palpating the carotid pulse or by looking for the QRS complex on the electrocardiogram (ECG) monitor's oscilloscope.

All systolic murmurs occur between the first heart sound (S_1) and the second heart sound (S_2) during ventricular systole; this is the interval between the QRS complex and the T wave on the ECG waveform. All diastolic murmurs occur between S_2 and S_1 during ventricular diastole; this is the interval between the T wave and the next QRS complex on the ECG waveform.

Murmurs are further classified according to their timing in the phases of the cardiac cycle. For example, a murmur can be described as "holosystolic," meaning it's present throughout systole, or as "early systolic," "midsystolic," "late systolic," or "diastolic."

Murmur configurations

Crescendo/decrescendo
(diamond-shaped)
- Begins softly, peaks sharply, and then fades
- Examples: Pulmonic stenosis, aortic stenosis, mitral valve prolapse, mitral stenosis

Decrescendo
- Starts loudly and then gradually diminishes
- Examples: Aortic insufficiency, pulmonic insufficiency

Pansystolic
(holosystolic or plateau-shaped)
- Is uniform from beginning to end
- Examples: Mitral or tricuspid regurgitation

Crescendo
- Begins softly and then gradually increases
- Examples: Tricuspid stenosis, mitral valve prolapse

Configuration

The last murmur characteristic, configuration, refers to the shape or pattern of a murmur's sound as recorded on a phonocardiogram. The configuration usually is defined by changes in the murmur's intensity during systole or diastole and is determined by blood flow pressure gradients. For example:

- A crescendo murmur gradually increases in intensity as the pressure gradient increases.
- A decrescendo murmur gradually decreases in intensity as the pressure gradient decreases.
- A crescendo-decrescendo murmur first increases in intensity as the pressure gradient increases, and then decreases in intensity as the pressure gradient decreases; it's also known as a *diamond-shaped murmur.*
- A plateau-shaped murmur remains equal in intensity throughout the murmur. (See *Murmur configurations.*)

9 Systolic murmurs

In a heart that's functioning normally, as ventricular pressures rise at the beginning of systole, the mitral and tricuspid valves close. Then, for a brief time during isovolumic contraction, while the aortic and pulmonic valves are still closed, ventricular pressures rise sharply. When the pressure in both ventricles is high enough, the aortic and pulmonic valves open and blood is ejected from the ventricles into the aorta and the pulmonary artery. Valves that are functioning properly facilitate this unidirectional blood flow.

Systolic murmurs can occur when these valves have a defect. All systolic murmurs occur during ventricular systole between the first heart sound (S_1) and the second heart sound (S_2). Aortic or pulmonic outlet abnormalities may generate forward systolic ejection murmurs (SEMs). When the mitral or tricuspid valve is involved, backward (or regurgitant) murmurs may occur.

KNOW-HOW *Usually, a systolic murmur is high-pitched (representing the high pressure and high velocity of blood during ventricular ejection); therefore, it's heard best using the diaphragm of the stethoscope.*

Innocent and pathologic murmurs

During ventricular systole, the rapid ejection of blood from the ventricles causes turbulent blood flow that can produce innocent systolic murmurs. **(SOUND 27)** These murmurs, which can be described as benign or functional, are considered normal in most people. They can be caused simply by normal physiologic conditions, such as pregnancy, which requires a high volume of blood circulating throughout the body.

Quite commonly, innocent murmurs (also called *Still's murmurs*) can also be heard in infants or children and in thin-chested people. These murmurs aren't caused by structural abnormalities of the heart.

About half of people older than age 50 have innocent systolic murmurs. They're more common in women and in patients with hypertension. These systolic murmurs may not be so innocent when they occur in the presence of certain disease processes, such as anemia, fever, and thyrotoxicosis, because they can cause high-flow situations in which the accompanying systolic murmur isn't related to a cardiac defect.

The quality of innocent SEMs is variable. Other characteristics include soft intensity (less than a grade III/IV), short duration, distinctive start and end points, early diastolic timing and ending well before a normal S_2 split, and crescendo-decrescendo configuration.
(SOUND 27)

Pathologic systolic murmurs are usually caused by:
- stenosis of the aortic valve or pulmonic valve
- insufficiency of the mitral valve or tricuspid valve
- interventricular septal defects.

A person may be born with a congenital defect or may acquire a defect from such secondary conditions as rheumatic heart disease or idiopathic calcification of the valves. Because of the progressive nature of valve defects (for example, aortic stenosis), the timing and other characteristics of a systolic murmur can help to determine the severity of the disease.

When determining whether a systolic murmur is innocent or pathologic, it's important to consider the patient's history and symptoms and the results of pertinent examinations and tests, including a chest X-ray, electrocardiogram (ECG), and echocardiography. Most innocent systolic murmurs occur in early systole or midsystole.

Classifying systolic murmurs

Systolic murmurs are classified as either ejection or regurgitant. SEMs are audible only during part of systole; that is, they start after S_1 and end before S_2 begins. (See *Auscultating for SEMs,* page 104.) Because these murmurs are caused by aortic or pulmonary abnormalities, they're divided into two categories: pulmonic SEMs and aortic SEMs.

Auscultating for SEMs

To determine whether a murmur intensifies, listen at the murmur's border. Usually, you'll hear a systolic ejection murmur (SEM) best along the left sternal border and, sometimes, over the aortic and mitral areas, as shown here.

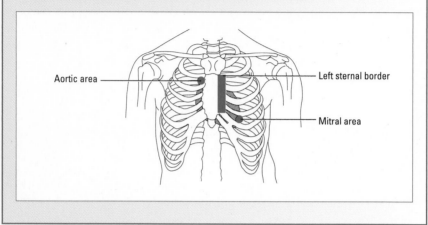

Regurgitant murmurs are audible throughout all of systole—that is, they start with S_1 and end with S_2.

KNOW-HOW *An SEM has a medium pitch that's heard best with the diaphragm of the stethoscope. An SEM's intensity can be increased by movements that increase blood volume or ejection velocity, such as having the patient raise his legs from a recumbent position, exercise briefly, or cough a few times.*

Pulmonic systolic ejection murmurs

Pulmonic SEMs are caused by right ventricular outflow tract (RVOT) obstruction. RVOT obstruction stems from pulmonic stenosis, which is narrowing of the artery or valve. It may be supravalvular, valvular, or subvalvular. Regardless of location, the outflow obstruction causes turbulent blood flow that produces a midsystolic ejection murmur.

The murmur begins early in systole—after S_1 and the opening of the diseased pulmonic valve. It ends before the S_2 closure component of the diseased pulmonic valve. This murmur typically has a crescendo-decrescendo configuration that peaks in intensity in early systole,

Understanding supravalvular pulmonic stenosis murmurs

Supravalvular pulmonic stenosis murmurs occur in the area slightly above the pulmonic artery, as shown here.

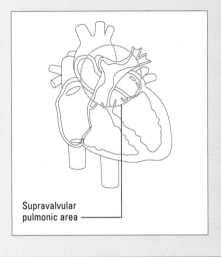

Supravalvular
pulmonic area

midsystole, or late systole, depending on the severity of the obstruction.

Supravalvular pulmonic stenosis murmurs

Supravalvular pulmonic stenosis, or pulmonary artery branch stenosis, is a type of RVOT obstruction that occurs above the pulmonic valve. (See *Understanding supravalvular pulmonic stenosis murmurs*.) Rarely, the murmur is accompanied by a pulmonic ejection sound (PES). **(SOUND 28)** Supravalvular pulmonic stenosis commonly occurs with rubella syndrome or Williams syndrome (unusual facial appearance, mental retardation, hypercalcemia).

Sound characteristics

Supravalvular pulmonic stenosis murmurs usually can be heard over much of the thorax. (See *Auscultating for supravalvular pulmonic stenosis murmurs, page 106.*)

Other characteristics include:
- variable intensity and duration
- medium pitch that's heard best with the diaphragm of the stethoscope

Auscultating for supravalvular pulmonic stenosis murmurs

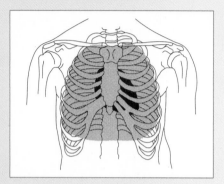

You can auscultate for supravalvular pulmonic stenosis murmurs over much of the thorax, as highlighted in this illustration.

Supravalvular pulmonic stenosis murmurs on PCG and ECG

A supravalvular pulmonic stenosis murmur has a crescendo-decrescendo configuration. The murmur starts just after the QRS complex and ends before the T wave begins, as shown in this phonocardiogram (PCG) and electrocardiogram (ECG) representation.

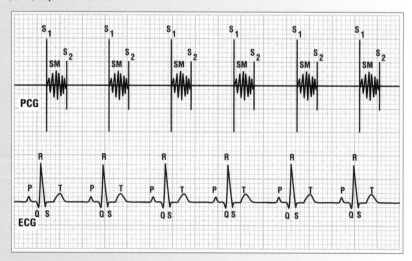

Understanding valvular pulmonic stenosis murmurs

The pulmonic valvular area, as shown here, produces a valvular pulmonic stenosis murmur.

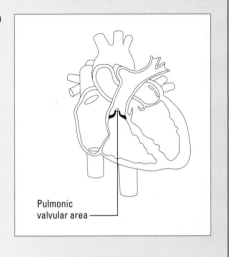

Pulmonic valvular area

- harsh quality
- systolic timing starting after S_1 and ending before a normal S_2 split (see *Supravalvular pulmonic stenosis murmurs on PCG and ECG*)
- location on an ECG starting just after the QRS complex begins and ending just before the T wave ends
- crescendo-decrescendo configuration that's occasionally continuous. **(SOUND 28)**

Valvular pulmonic stenosis murmurs

A valvular pulmonic stenosis (or pulmonic valve stenosis) murmur is the most common type and accounts for more than 90% of pulmonic stenosis cases. It results from congenital pulmonic valvular stenosis and commonly occurs with other congenital heart defects. (See *Understanding valvular pulmonic stenosis murmurs.*) In mild pulmonic valve stenosis, S_1 is normal. The murmur begins after S_1 with a right-sided PES as the pulmonic valve abruptly stops opening. Remember, the PES is the only right-sided heart sound that increases in intensity during expiration and becomes less audible during inspiration. The murmur intensifies after the PES and peaks in midsystole; then it begins to fade. It ends before S_2. **(SOUND 29)**

Auscultating for valvular pulmonic stenosis murmurs

When auscultating for valvular pulmonic stenosis murmurs, place your stethoscope over the pulmonic area at the left sternal border, as shown here.

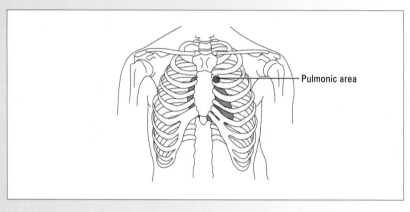

Pulmonic area

In severe valvular pulmonic stenosis, the pressure gradient across the pulmonic valve increases. An increased pressure gradient causes the PES to occur earlier; it may even fuse with S_1. Right ventricular ejection time is also prolonged. As a result, the murmur has a longer crescendo and the intensity peaks later in systole. The prolonged right ventricular ejection time also causes a delay, creating a wide S_2 split. Usually, as the stenosis becomes more severe, the murmur's duration lengthens and its configuration becomes more asymmetrical.

Sound characteristics

Valvular pulmonic stenosis murmurs are heard best near the base of the heart, over the pulmonic area. (See *Auscultating for valvular pulmonic stenosis murmurs.*)

Other characteristics include:
- radiation toward the left neck or the left shoulder
- soft intensity that becomes louder with a palpable thrill toward the left neck and shoulder as stenosis becomes more severe
- short duration that increases as stenosis worsens
- medium pitch that's heard best with the diaphragm of the stethoscope

Understanding subvalvular pulmonic stenosis murmurs

The area below the pulmonary artery produces subvalvular pulmonic stenosis murmurs.

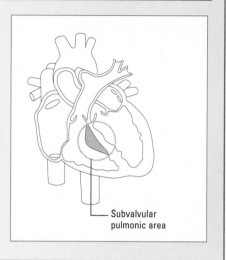

Subvalvular pulmonic area

- harsh quality
- midsystolic timing ending before a normal S_2 split
- accompanying PES that diminishes or disappears with inspiration
- location on an ECG beginning after the QRS complex and ending before the end of the T wave
- crescendo-decrescendo configuration
- diamond shape (mild valvular pulmonic stenosis murmur)
- kite shape (severe pulmonic valvular stenosis murmur).

(SOUND 29)

Subvalvular pulmonic stenosis murmurs

When an RVOT obstruction is subvalvular, or beneath the pulmonic valve, a midsystolic ejection murmur sounds the same as a pulmonic valvular stenosis murmur. (See *Understanding subvalvular pulmonic stenosis murmurs.*) However, this type of murmur isn't started by a PES. **(SOUND 30)** Subvalvular pulmonic stenosis is uncommon and linked to ventricular septal defects (VSDs) such as tetralogy of Fallot. When the subvalvular obstruction occurs with a VSD, the murmur is more complex.

Auscultating for subvalvular pulmonic stenosis murmurs

To listen for subvalvular pulmonic stenosis murmurs, place your stethoscope over the pulmonic area and over Erb's point, as shown here.

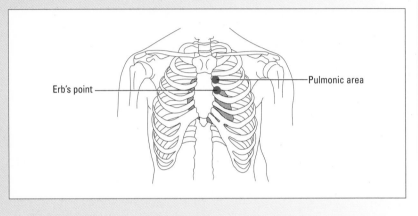

Erb's point

Pulmonic area

Sound characteristics

Subvalvular pulmonic stenosis murmurs are usually heard best over the pulmonic area and over Erb's point. They commonly radiate toward the left side of the neck, the left shoulder, or both. (See *Auscultating for subvalvular pulmonic stenosis murmurs.*)

Other characteristics include:

- soft intensity that becomes louder as stenosis worsens
- short duration that also increases as stenosis worsens
- medium pitch that's heard best with the diaphragm of the stethoscope
- harsh quality
- midsystolic timing starting after S_1 and ending before a normal S_2 split
- location on an ECG starting after the QRS complex and ending before the end of the T wave **(SOUND 30)**
- not initiated by a PES
- crescendo-decrescendo configuration.

Aortic systolic ejection murmurs

Aortic SEMs are caused by left ventricular outflow tract (LVOT) ob-structions. LVOT obstructions are associated with aortic stenosis, which is a narrowing of the aorta through which the blood leaves the heart. Other causes of aortic SEMs include aortic dilation, aortic valve sclerosis, and increased aortic flow. Aortic stenosis may be supravalvular, valvular, or subvalvular. Regardless of location, the outflow obstruction causes turbulent blood flow that produces a midsystolic ejection murmur.

The murmur begins early in systole—after S_1 and the opening of the diseased aortic valve. It ends before the S_2 closure component of the diseased aortic valve. This murmur typically has a crescendo-decrescendo configuration that peaks in intensity in early systole, midsystole, or late systole, depending on the obstruction's severity.

Supravalvular aortic stenosis murmurs

Supravalvular aortic stenosis murmurs are usually congenital and are caused by aortic coarctation and fixed supravalvular stenosis. (See *Understanding supravalvular aortic stenosis murmurs.*)

Understanding supravalvular aortic stenosis murmurs

Supravalvular aortic stenosis murmurs affect the ascending aorta by creating either an hourglass-shaped internal constriction or a diffuse narrowing of the area.

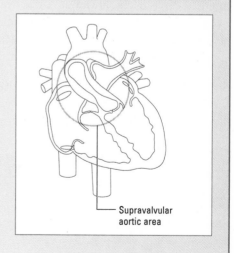

Supravalvular
aortic area

Auscultating for supravalvular aortic stenosis murmurs

When auscultating for supravalvular aortic stenosis murmurs, place your stethoscope over the base of the heart at the right 1st intercostal space, over the aortic area, and over the suprasternal notch, as shown here.

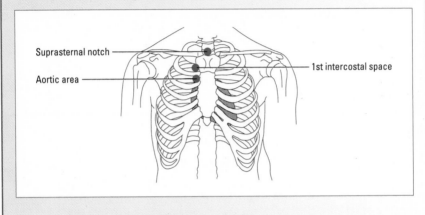

Other causes of supravalvular aortic stenosis murmurs are rare but may include fibrous membranes and fibromuscular ridges above the aortic sinuses. These causes may produce a murmur similar to that heard with aortic valvular stenosis but louder, without an aortic ejection sound (AES), and heard best over the suprasternal area, aortic area, or right first intercostal space. **(SOUND 31)**

Sound characteristics

Supravalvular aortic stenosis murmurs are usually heard best near the base of the heart over the right first intercostal space, over the aortic area, and over the suprasternal notch. (See *Auscultating for supravalvular aortic stenosis murmurs.*)

Other characteristics include:
- radiation toward the right side of the neck, the right shoulder, or both
- typically grade III/VI to IV/VI intensity, decreasing in patients with left-sided heart failure
- increased duration as stenosis worsens
- medium pitch that's heard equally well with the diaphragm or bell of the stethoscope
- rough quality

Understanding valvular aortic stenosis murmurs

In valvular aortic stenosis, the aorta may have structural abnormalities, such as abnormal cusp formations, or calcification may occur.

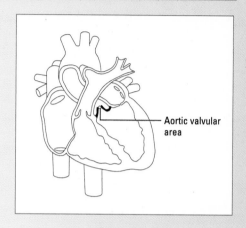

Aortic valvular area

- midsystolic timing that ends before the normal S_2 split
- no associated AES
- location on an ECG starting after the QRS complex and ending before the end of the T wave
- crescendo-decrescendo configuration (when an LVOT obstruction is above the aortic valve or supravalvular). **(SOUND 31)**

Valvular aortic stenosis murmurs

Valvular aortic stenosis, most commonly known as *aortic valve stenosis,* may be congenital or may result from degenerative or rheumatic heart disease. (See *Understanding valvular aortic stenosis murmurs.*) If it results from rheumatic heart disease, the mitral valve usually is also affected. Aortic stenosis produces an SEM that begins after S_1 and ends before S_2. **(SOUND 32)** (See *Responding to aortic stenosis,* page 114.)

After S_1, left ventricular pressure rises. The stenotic aortic valve halts its opening motion and produces a loud AES that's heard best near the apex of the heart over the mitral area. The AES is followed by the murmur, which gradually intensifies until midsystole to late systole and then fades, ending before S_2.

Sound characteristics

Valvular aortic stenosis murmurs are usually heard best near the base of the heart over the aortic area, over Erb's point, near the apex of the

CASE CLIP

Responding to aortic stenosis

Mr. C., a 42-year-old man, presented to the urgent care center for evaluation of increased shortness of breath, intermittent chest pain with exertion, and one episode of syncope while working. On interview at the urgent care center, Mr. C. told the staff that he hasn't seen a doctor for more than 10 years, takes no prescription medication, and occasionally uses acetaminophen for headaches. He reports being healthy most of his life, experienced normal childhood illnesses, and a history of rheumatic fever as a child. He thought his current symptoms were related to working outside in the heat as a carpenter, however, after they persisted he finally agreed at his wife's insistence to get a checkup.

Assessment revealed a well-developed white male in no acute distress. Mr C.'s vital signs were:
- temperature: 97.8° F (36.6° C)
- heart rate (HR): 64 beats/minute
- respiratory rate: 8 breaths/minute and unlabored
- blood pressure (BP): 152/90 mm Hg.

He was alert and oriented. Breath sounds revealed bibasilar crackles. No jugular vein distention was present, however 1+ pitting lower limb edema was noted. On assessment of heart sounds, he was noted to have a holosystolic harsh murmur over the right sternal border aortic area with radiation to the neck, which was graded IV/VI on the I to VI scale for grading heart murmurs. An electrocardiogram (ECG) revealed a normal sinus rhythm.

Based on physical examination, the urgent care provider suspected aortic stenosis and ordered a two-dimensional Doppler echocardiogram which confirmed moderate-to-severe aortic stenosis. Based on the results of the echocardiogram, before discharge from the urgent care center, an appointment was made for Mr. C. with a cardiovascular surgeon for the next day. As part of his discharge instructions from the urgent care center, Mr. C. was told that if he experienced changes in his symptoms or had another episode of chest pain, he should call 911 and go to the emergency department immediately.

After the surgeon examined Mr. C., he found his BP remained elevated at 166/84 mm Hg and his HR was tachycardic at 110 beats/minute and irregular. Another ECG was performed and showed frequent premature ventricular contractions. The surgeon reviewed the echocardiogram results and recommended valve replacement based on Mr. C.'s echocardiogram, angina, and heart failure symptoms. Before surgery, a cardiac catheterization was performed to further assess coronary artery perfusion. If the angiogram had shown coronary artery disease, a bypass or angioplasty would have been done before the surgery.

Mr. C. did well after surgery with full recovery expected and the ability to return to work. Because of the mechanical valve, he will have to remain on warfarin anticoagulation therapy for life.

Auscultating for valvular aortic stenosis murmurs

When auscultating for valvular aortic stenosis murmurs, place your stethoscope over the aortic area, the mitral area, over Erb's point, or over the suprasternal notch, as highlighted here.

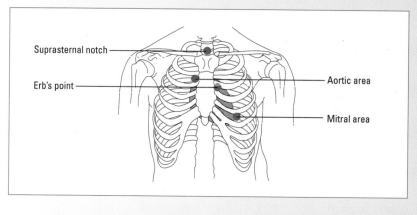

heart over the mitral area, or over the suprasternal notch. (See *Auscultating for valvular aortic stenosis murmurs*.) In older adults, these murmurs aren't as easy to find.

Other characteristics include:

■ radiation toward the right side of the neck, the right shoulder, or both

■ possible palpable thrill over the aortic area and neck

■ varying intensity from soft grade II/VI to rough grade IV/VI sound (typically grade III/VI to IV/VI intensity, decreasing in patients with left-sided heart failure)

■ increasing duration as stenosis worsens

■ medium pitch that's heard equally well with the diaphragm or bell of the stethoscope

■ rough quality that becomes harsher and louder with worsening stenosis

■ midsystolic timing

■ an AES heard shortly after S_1 (when present); AES following murmur, ending before a normal S_2 split

■ severe stenosis (if an S_4 is heard in a patient younger than age 40)

Understanding subvalvular aortic stenosis murmurs

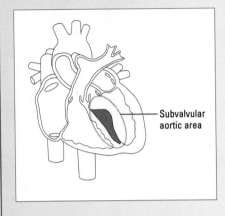

Subvalvular aortic stenosis murmurs may result from a fibrous ring obstruction below the aortic valve or an abnormal hypertrophy of the septum.

Subvalvular aortic area

- location on an ECG waveform starting after the QRS complex and ending before the end of the T wave
- crescendo-decrescendo configuration. **(SOUND 32)**

Subvalvular aortic stenosis murmurs

A subvalvular aortic outflow obstruction may be caused by fixed subaortic stenosis (which may present as a long, fixed segment or a short, fibrous ring) or hypertrophic cardiomyopathy, a genetic cardiac disorder. **(SOUND 33)** This obstruction is produced by asymmetrical hypertrophy or thickening of the septum and abnormal anterior motion of the mitral valve leaflets during systole. (See *Understanding subvalvular aortic stenosis murmurs*.)

Sound characteristics

Subvalvular aortic stenosis murmurs are usually heard best near the apex of the heart over the mitral and tricuspid areas. (See *Auscultating for subvalvular aortic stenosis murmurs*.)
    Other characteristics include:

- usually no radiation toward the base, right side of the neck, or right shoulder
- typically grade III/VI to IV/VI intensity that increases as stenosis worsens
- variable duration

Auscultating for subvalvular aortic stenosis murmurs

Subvalvular aortic stenosis murmurs are best heard over the apex of the heart. Place your stethoscope over the tricuspid and mitral areas, shown here.

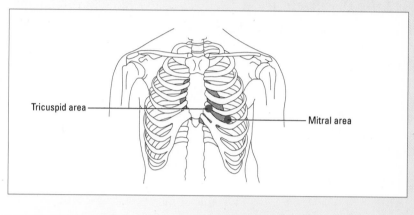

Tricuspid area

Mitral area

■ medium pitch that's heard equally well with the bell or diaphragm of the stethoscope
■ harsh or rough quality
■ midsystolic timing peaking in midsystole and ending before a normal S_2 split or a paradoxical S_2 split
■ location on an ECG starting after the QRS complex and ending before the end of the T wave
■ crescendo-decrescendo configuration. **(SOUND 33)**

Differentiating subvalvular and valvular aortic stenosis murmurs

Because subvalvular and valvular aortic murmurs have similar characteristics, they may be difficult to differentiate. Here are some tips for distinguishing between them.
■ A subvalvular hypertrophic cardiomyopathic murmur becomes louder during Valsalva's maneuver, whereas a valvular aortic stenosis murmur doesn't. Performing Valsalva's maneuver or having the patient quickly stand up decreases venous return and left ventricular filling; this makes the left ventricle smaller, the obstruction more severe, and the subvalvular hypertrophic obstructive cardiomyopathic murmur louder.

- Having the patient squat increases peripheral vascular resistance and left ventricular filling; this maneuver decreases the pressure gradient across the aortic valve and decreases or obliterates the subvalvular hypertrophic obstructive cardiomyopathic murmur.

Systolic insufficiency murmurs

There are three types of systolic insufficiency murmurs:
- tricuspid insufficiency murmur
- mitral insufficiency murmur
- VSD murmur.

An abnormality of either the tricuspid or mitral valve may result in backward turbulent blood flow during systole, so blood moves in the opposite direction of its normal unidirectional flow. Blood regurgitates through a defective, incompetent tricuspid or mitral valve into the left or right atrium, resulting in what's commonly called *tricuspid valve insufficiency* or *mitral valve insufficiency,* respectively.

An incompetent valve may be caused by a primary valvular disorder or may develop secondary to dysfunction of the valve's supporting structures, as in a VSD. A hole in the ventricular septum causes oxygenated and deoxygenated blood to mix and causes a VSD murmur.

The regurgitant murmurs heard in patients with these valve disorders may be in early or late systole, or they may be holosystolic. Early

Understanding tricuspid insufficiency murmurs

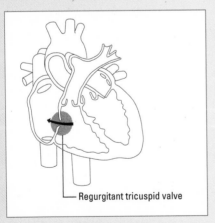

Tricuspid insufficiency murmurs commonly are caused by right ventricular dilation and an abnormal tricuspid valve, as shown here.

Regurgitant tricuspid valve

systolic murmurs have a crescendo-decrescendo configuration, late systolic murmurs have either a crescendo or crescendo-decrescendo configuration, and holosystolic murmurs have a plateau shape.

Tricuspid insufficiency murmurs

Tricuspid insufficiency murmurs, also called *tricuspid regurgitation murmurs,* most commonly result from right ventricular dilation, which usually is caused by mitral valve disease or left-sided heart failure but may also be caused by pulmonary disease.

Occasionally, tricuspid insufficiency murmurs result from congenital valve malformation or from infective endocarditis, a right ventricular infarction, or trauma to the valve or its supporting structures. (See *Understanding tricuspid insufficiency murmurs.*)

A tricuspid insufficiency murmur can also be heard in a patient with a transvenous pacemaker because the pacemaker lead interferes with tricuspid valve closure, creating a tricuspid insufficiency type murmur. The T_1 (tricuspid valve closure) intensity may be increased, normal, or decreased. **(SOUND 34)**

Sound characteristics

Tricuspid insufficiency murmurs usually are heard best over the tricuspid area; in some patients, they're heard only during inspiration. (See *Auscultating for tricuspid insufficiency murmurs.*)

Auscultating for tricuspid insufficiency murmurs

To auscultate for tricuspid insufficiency murmurs, place the stethoscope over the tricuspid area, as shown here.

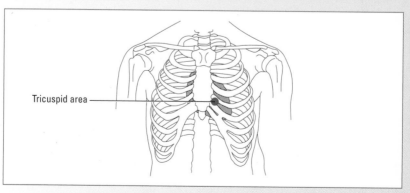

Tricuspid area

Understanding mitral insufficiency murmurs

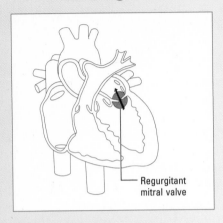

Mitral insufficiency murmurs are caused by an abnormality of the mitral valve, as shown here, or the left ventricle.

Regurgitant mitral valve

Other characteristics include:
- radiation to the right of the sternum
- soft intensity that increases during deep inspiration
- increasing intensity during inspiration (regardless of the murmur's cause) because venous return and right ventricular filling are increased, creating higher pressure gradients during systole
- long duration
- medium pitch that's heard best with the diaphragm of the stethoscope
- scratchy or blowing quality
- rarely accompanied by a systolic thrill
- no correlation between intensity or timing in systole and the severity of the insufficiency
- systolic timing lasting from S_1 to S_2
- location on an ECG waveform starting just after the QRS complex and ending after the T wave
- holosystolic character
- plateau shape. **(SOUND 34)**

KNOW-HOW A tricuspid insufficiency murmur is louder during inspiration. In some patients, this is the only time the murmur is audible. To enhance the murmur, have the patient breathe through his mouth slowly, quietly, and more deeply while sitting or standing. Caution the patient not to hold his breath because this negates the maneuver's effect. Remember, however, that right ventricular filling may be limited with

Auscultating for mitral insufficiency murmurs

For all types of mitral insufficiency murmurs, including holosystolic murmurs, acute mitral insufficiency murmurs, and mitral valve prolapse murmurs, place the stethoscope over the mitral area, as shown here.

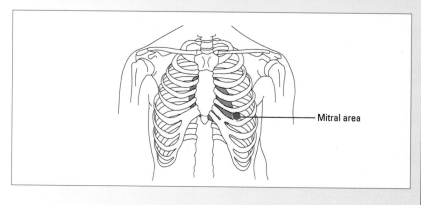

Mitral area

inspiration if a tricuspid insufficiency murmur is secondary to right-sided heart failure; consequently, the murmur may not intensify during deep breathing.

Mitral insufficiency murmurs

Mitral insufficiency murmurs, also called *mitral regurgitation murmurs,* may be caused by congenital or acquired abnormalities of the mitral valve leaflets, the valve's supporting structures, or the left ventricle. An incompetent mitral valve causes backward blood flow during systole. The increased pressure at the aortic valve facilitates regurgitation of blood through the incompetent mitral valve into the low-pressure left atrium, producing a mitral insufficiency murmur. **(SOUND 35)** (See *Understanding mitral insufficiency murmurs.*)

Sound characteristics

Mitral insufficiency murmurs are best heard over the mitral area. (See *Auscultating for mitral insufficiency murmurs.*)
Other characteristics include:

■ appearance in early systole, midsystole, or late systole or holosystolic

■ quality, duration, and radiation varying with extent, duration, and location of the disease process

■ usually associated with mild to moderate insufficiency (if late).

Holosystolic mitral insufficiency murmurs

Holosystolic mitral insufficiency murmurs can be caused by:
- the effects of rheumatic heart disease on the mitral valve
- mitral valve prolapse
- left ventricular dilation
- papillary muscle dysfunction.

A loud S_3 usually accompanies moderate to severe mitral insufficiency; this sound isn't related to ventricular failure but to the increased left ventricular volume in early diastole.

Sound characteristics

Holosystolic mitral insufficiency murmurs are usually heard best near the heart's apex over the mitral area.

 KNOW-HOW *Holosystolic mitral insufficiency murmurs can usually be heard regardless of the patient's position, but grade I/VI to II/VI murmurs may be heard better with the patient in the partial left lateral recumbent position or after exercise.*

Other characteristics include:
- radiation to the axillae or posteriorly over the lung bases
- variable intensity that usually isn't affected by respiration but may be somewhat diminished during inspiration
- long duration
- medium to high pitch that's heard best with the diaphragm of the stethoscope
- accompanying systolic apical thrill
- blowing quality
- systolic timing from S_1 to S_2
- location on an ECG just after the QRS complex to the end of the T wave
- holosystolic character
- plateau shape. **(SOUND 35)**

Acute mitral insufficiency murmurs

Acute mitral insufficiency murmurs are less common than chronic mitral insufficiency murmurs. Resulting from rupture of the chordae tendineae, papillary muscle, or both, these murmurs occasionally are caused by myocardial infarction but also may be caused by severe damage to the mitral valve from trauma or infection. (See *Responding to acute mitral regurgitation.*)

CASE CLIP

Responding to acute mitral regurgitation

Mr. B. was a 62-year-old male who presented to the urgent care center after experiencing chest pain about 2 days earlier while out working in the fields on his tractor. He described the discomfort as a crushing sensation in the middle of his chest, which lasted about 2 hours. He blamed it on indigestion after eating a hot dog with chili for lunch that day. However, over the next 2 days, he experienced increasing shortness of breath. The next day, he didn't go out to work because the significant effort it took him to get dressed had frightened him. In the past, he had been relatively healthy except for being treated for hypertension. There was a notable family history of heart disease in his father and two brothers who all had myocardial infarctions (MIs) in their late 50s.

Assessment revealed a white male who appeared his stated age, well-developed, alert, and oriented. He did appear to be in mild distress with increasingly labored breathing. Mr. B.'s vital signs were:

- temperature: 98.9° F (37.2° C)
- heart rate (HR): 78 beats/minute
- respiratory rate (RR): 24 breaths/minute
- blood pressure (BP): 120/58 mm Hg.

Bibasilar crackles were noted. No jugular vein distention or edema were noted. His abdomen was soft, nondistended, and nontender. Auscultation of the heart revealed a holosystolic grade III/VI murmur heard best over the mitral area. An electrocardiogram showed changes consistent with an inferior wall MI. A subsequent echocardiogram showed a papillary muscle rupture.

Based on assessment findings, Mr. B. was diagnosed with acute mitral insufficiency secondary to papillary muscle rupture. The underlying etiology was considered to be an acute MI on the day of his initial symptoms. A troponin level was drawn and an elevated result validated the diagnosis. Mr. B. was considered a high-risk patient and the local emergency medical service was contacted to transport him to the area hospital. Before transfer his vital signs were:

- HR: 104 beats/minute
- RR: 22 breaths/minute
- BP: increased to 140/92 mm Hg
- pulse oximetry: 95%.

An I.V. of normal saline solution was started and Mr. B. was given 5 mg of I.V. lopressor before the transfer. He was admitted for emergency surgery for mitral valve replacement as well as angioplasty of the right coronary and circumflex arteries.

Mr. B fully recovered after surgery and was able to return to work. Because of the mechanical valve, he will have to remain on anticoagulation therapy for life.

An acute mitral insufficiency murmur is a decrescendo murmur that begins with mitral valve closure. **(SOUND 36)** Its intensity decreases as ventricular and atrial pressures equalize during late systole. An S_4 is usually heard in acute mitral insufficiency.

Sound characteristics

Acute mitral insufficiency murmurs usually are heard best near the heart's apex over the mitral area.

Other characteristics include:
- loud intensity (grade IV/VI to VI/VI if the murmur results from rupture of the chordae tendineae)
- accompanying systolic thrill
- medium to long duration
- high pitch that's heard best with the diaphragm of the stethoscope
- musical quality
- systolic timing
- location on an ECG starting just after the QRS complex and ending just after the T wave
- commonly a holosystolic character and wedge shape (the wedge shape has a steeper decrescendo configuration). **(SOUND 36)**

Mitral valve prolapse murmurs

Mitral valve prolapse is one of the most common valvular abnormalities in adults. The murmur of mitral valve prolapse usually appears in late systole and is either isolated or accompanied by a nonejection midsystolic click (a click caused by the mitral valve prolapsing and ballooning up into the left atrium). Consequently, a mitral valve prolapse murmur sometimes is called a *click-murmur syndrome.* **(SOUND 37)** (See *Responding to mitral valve prolapse.*)

Sound characteristics

Mitral valve prolapse murmurs usually are heard best near the apex of the heart over the mitral area. (See *Tips for hearing mitral valve prolapse murmurs,* page 126.)

Other characteristics include:
- soft intensity (grade II/VI to III/VI)
- short duration
- high pitch that's heard best with the diaphragm of the stethoscope
- musical quality (when loud, can be described as a whoop or a honk)
- late systolic timing (may be holosystolic)

CASE CLIP

Responding to mitral valve prolapse

Ms. A., a 22-year-old woman, presented to her practitioner for complaints of chest pain, occasional shortness of breath, and the sensation of a racing heart. Her symptoms would last seconds to minutes, often occurring during a workout session. In general, her health had been good and the only medication she was taking was daily birth control pills. There was no family history of cardiac disease. She was a nondrinker, nonsmoker, and denied illicit drug use. She was single and had no children. Her symptoms started 6 months earlier, but gradually increased in frequency causing her enough concern to seek medical evaluation.

On assessment, she was alert and oriented and in no acute distress. She was well-nourished and well-developed. On examination, her vital signs were:

- temperature: 98.6° F (37° C)
- heart rate: 62 beats/minute
- respiratory rate: 24 breaths/minute
- blood pressure: 94/66 mm Hg.

On auscultation, her lungs were found to be clear. Her abdomen was flat, soft, and nontender. There was no thyroidmegaly present. There was no edema or jugular vein distention. On assessment of heart sounds, her practitioner noted a midsystolic click with a grade I/VI systolic murmur. An electrocardiogram was obtained and showed ST-T wave depression in the inferior leads I, II, and aV$_F$. The practitioner suspected mitral valve prolapse which was confirmed by obtaining an echocardiogram. Mild mitral insufficiency was noted as well, explaining the systolic murmur that was noted.

Many patients with mitral valve prolapse are asymptomatic, however, as in Ms. A.'s case, they can present with such symptoms as atypical chest pain, fatigue, dyspnea and, most commonly, palpitations secondary to arrhythmias. Most patients don't require treatment. However, in symptomatic patients such as Ms. A., they typically respond well with the use of beta-adrenergic blockers, which diminish the recurrence of arrhythmias.

As part of Ms. A.'s patient education before her discharge she was advised to return to her cardiologist yearly and to inform her dentist of her mitral valve prolapse, so that prophylactic antibiotics can be administered before she has dental work.

- location on an ECG coinciding with the T wave and ending just after the T wave
- crescendo or crescendo-decrescendo configuration. **(SOUND 37)**

KNOW-HOW

Tips for hearing mitral valve prolapse murmurs

Here are some tips for improving your auscultation of mitral valve prolapse murmurs.

Positioning for timing
Ask the patient to stand; which decreases left ventricular volume. This allows a mitral valve prolapse murmur to be heard earlier in systole, to be louder, and to last longer. Having the patient squat increases left ventricular volume, which causes the murmur to be heard later in systole.

Disease-dependent direction
The direction in which the mitral valve prolapse murmur is transmitted across the chest wall depends on the disease process. For example, if the mitral valve's posterior leaflet is involved, blood flow might be directed more anteriorly and medially. As a result, the murmur would be transmitted toward the heart's base and heard best over the aortic area and along the left sternal edge. If the anterior leaflet is incompetent, blood flow is directed posteriorly against the posterior left atrial wall, and the murmur is transmitted toward the left axilla and back.

Understanding VSD murmurs

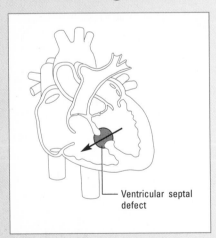

Ventricular septal defect

A ventricular septal defect (VSD) murmur occurs when a defect or opening in the ventricular septum allows blood to mix between the right and left ventricles, as shown here.

Auscultating for VSD murmurs

To hear a ventricular septal defect (VSD) murmur, place the stethoscope over the lower left sternal border. If the murmur is loud, you may be able to hear it over the entire precordium. These areas are shown here.

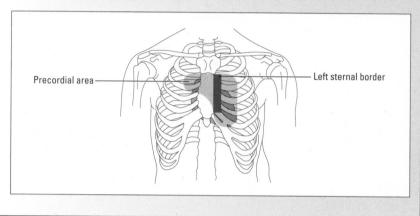

Precordial area — Left sternal border

Ventricular septal defect murmurs

A VSD is an opening, usually in the membranous portion of the ventricular septum that allows direct communication between the ventricles. (See *Understanding VSD murmurs*.)

Usually, VSDs are congenital, appearing at birth. Typically, blood shunts from left to right because of higher pressures in the left ventricle.

Sound characteristics

The VSD murmur is heard over the lower left sternal border and, if loud, can be heard over the entire precordium. (See *Auscultating for VSD murmurs*.)

Other characteristics include:
- palpable thrill along the lower left sternal border
- holosystolic character
- widely split S_2 as the aortic valve closes early
- intensity and pitch that vary with the size of the VSD.

10 *Diastolic murmurs*

During auscultation, diastole is normally silent. You may, however, hear certain brief sounds that are also considered normal. These include the aortic component–pulmonic component (A_2–P_2) interval (as the aortic and pulmonic valves close) and a third heart sound (S_3) in a healthy person younger than age 20 (as the mitral and tricuspid valves open and the ventricles begin to fill).

Occasionally, you also may hear a fourth heart sound (S_4) as the atria contract at the end of diastole to pump blood into the ventricles. S_4—always an abnormal heart sound—is commonly heard in people with conditions that increase resistance to ventricular filling, such as a weak left ventricle.

A murmur heard during diastole is also considered abnormal. Unlike certain systolic murmurs, which can be innocent, diastolic murmurs almost always signal an underlying cardiac problem.

You can hear diastolic murmurs between the second heart sound (S_2) and the next first heart sound (S_1)—or, on an electrocardiogram (ECG) waveform, between the end of the T wave and the start of the QRS complex. When you hear a murmur, you first need to identify its timing. The timing is important information that can be used to help determine the murmur's cause.

Timing of diastolic murmurs

Diastolic murmurs are associated with ventricular relaxation and filling. They're described according to their timing during diastole. For example, a diastolic murmur may be described as early diastolic, middiastolic, late diastolic, or holodiastolic (occurring throughout diastole).

An early diastolic murmur starts in S_2 and peaks in the early phase of diastole. Because the aortic and pulmonic valves close at the start of diastole, an early diastolic murmur usually results from insufficiency of the aortic or pulmonic valve.

A middiastolic murmur occurs after S_2 and peaks in the middle phase of diastole. This is the time when the mitral and tricuspid valves open. Therefore, a middiastolic murmur usually signals stenosis of the mitral or tricuspid valve.

A late diastolic murmur also may result from mitral or tricuspid stenosis. The murmur starts and peaks in the latter half of diastole, although it may extend to the next S_1. For this reason, a late-diastolic murmur may also be called a *presystolic murmur.*

A holodiastolic, or pandiastolic, murmur starts with S_2 and extends throughout diastole. You'll typically hear this type of murmur in patients with patent ductus arteriosus or ventricular septal defects.

AGE ALERT Because S_3 and a holodiastolic murmur are both low-frequency sounds heard after the second heart sound, be careful not to confuse the two sounds during auscultation.

Depending on the patient's stage of life, an S_3 may be normal. S_3 results when decreased ventricular compliance accompanies increased ventricular volume during diastole. Because children and young adults normally have increased ventricular volume, an S_3 may be normal during these stages. Because of a high blood flow rate, a pregnant woman also may have an S_3. However, hearing a diastolic murmur during pregnancy is abnormal and warrants further attention.

In older adults, S_3 signals ventricular distress, an early sign of heart failure. S_3 is common in patients with coronary artery disease, cardiomyopathy, and patent ductus arteriosus.

Conditions causing diastolic murmurs

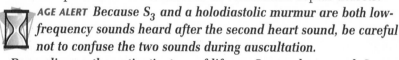

Because the ventricles relax and fill during diastole, a diastolic murmur typically results from an insufficiency of the aortic or pulmonic valve or stenosis of the mitral or tricuspid valve.

Aortic insufficiency

Aortic insufficiency, also called *aortic regurgitation,* may cause either an early diastolic murmur or a middiastolic murmur.

Understanding early diastolic aortic insufficiency murmurs

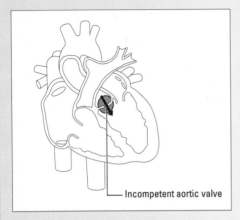

If the aortic valve fails to close properly, blood flows backward across the valve during diastole. This turbulent, backward flow across the incompetent valve, as shown here, produces the murmur.

Incompetent aortic valve

Early diastolic murmur

Pressure in the aorta normally exceeds pressure in the left ventricle at the start of diastole. If the aortic valve fails to close properly, blood flows backward (retrogrades) across the incompetent aortic valve.

This turbulent, backward flow produces an early diastolic murmur. In this instance, A_2 may sound normal or, if the patient has severe systemic hypertension, the sound may be accentuated. **(SOUND 38)** (See *Understanding early diastolic aortic insufficiency murmurs.*)

Commonly occurring with a systolic ejection murmur, this murmur may result from increased left ventricular stroke volume. Other possible causes include:
- rheumatic heart disease
- Marfan syndrome
- osteogenesis imperfecta
- dissecting aortic aneurysm.

Leakage around a prosthetic aortic valve may also produce an early diastolic murmur.

Sound characteristics

You'll hear an early diastolic aortic insufficiency murmur best when auscultating near the base of the heart (over the aortic and pulmonic

Auscultating for early diastolic murmurs in aortic insufficiency

To hear an early diastolic murmur caused by aortic insufficiency, listen near the base of the heart over the aortic and pulmonic areas, as shown here. You may also hear it by auscultating over Erb's point and the mitral area.

If the murmur is caused by aortic root dilation or a dissecting aneurysm of the ascending aorta, it may be louder along the right sternal border (between the 2nd and 4th intercostal spaces) than along the left sternal border.

If you're listening for the murmur in an elderly patient or one who has chronic obstructive pulmonary disease, try listening near the apex of the heart for best results. If the murmur is loud, you may be able to hear it over most of the precordium.

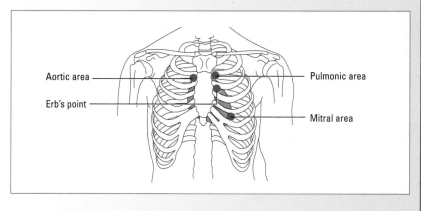

areas), over Erb's point, and near the apex of the heart (over the mitral area.) (See *Auscultating for early diastolic murmurs in aortic insufficiency*.)

Other characteristics include:

- soft intensity, so make sure to listen for it in a quiet environment
- high pitch, which is heard best with the diaphragm of the stethoscope
- a blowing or musical quality
- presence through most of diastole, starting with A_2
- location on an ECG starting after the T wave and ending just before the QRS complex
- decrescendo configuration. **(SOUND 38)**

Understanding Austin Flint murmurs

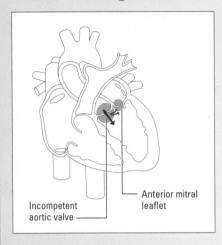

In cases of severe aortic insufficiency, blood regurgitated from the aortic valve can meet and interfere with blood flowing into the ventricle across the mitral valve. Blood flowing over the mitral valve becomes more turbulent and may make the mitral valve vibrate, which produces an Austin Flint murmur.

Incompetent aortic valve

Anterior mitral leaflet

KNOW-HOW *If you have trouble hearing an early diastolic aortic insufficiency murmur, have the patient perform maneuvers to increase aortic diastolic pressure. These maneuvers include having the patient sit down, lean forward, and hold his breath after exhaling; having him squat; or giving him handgrip exercises to perform.*

Middiastolic aortic (Austin Flint) murmur

If aortic insufficiency is severe, the backflow of blood from the aorta can interfere with the normal flow of blood across the mitral valve. The blood flowing across the mitral valve becomes more turbulent, causing the mitral valve to vibrate. In turn, this produces a middiastolic and presystolic rumbling murmur, also known as an *Austin Flint murmur.* **(SOUND 39)** (See *Understanding Austin Flint murmurs.*)

Sound characteristics
You'll hear an Austin Flint murmur best when auscultating near the apex of the heart, over the mitral area. (See *Auscultating for Austin Flint murmurs.*)

Other characteristics include:
■ a rumbling murmur
■ usually a soft intensity and low pitch, heard best with the bell of the stethoscope

Auscultating for Austin Flint murmurs

Because an Austin Flint murmur results from turbulent blood flow across the mitral valve, auscultate near the apex of the heart over the mitral area, as shown here, to hear the murmur clearly.

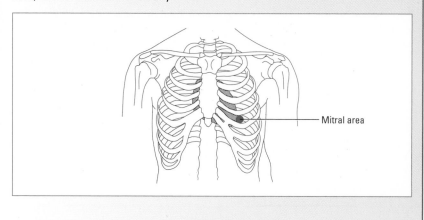

Mitral area

- location on an ECG just before the QRS complex
- crescendo configuration in the presystolic portion of the murmur and crescendo-decrescendo configuration in the middiastolic portion. **(SOUND 39)**

Pulmonic insufficiency

During systole, the right ventricle ejects blood into the low-pressure pulmonary circulation. Normally, the pulmonic valve prevents blood from returning to the right ventricle. In pulmonic insufficiency, blood flows backward from the pulmonary artery into the right ventricle.

A small amount of blood typically flows back across the valve in healthy adults, particularly in elderly people. However, an excessive backflow, or regurgitation, of blood can impair right ventricular function, leading to right-sided volume overload and heart failure.

Two types of pulmonic valve insufficiency murmurs may occur: Graham Steell's murmur and normal pressure pulmonic valve murmur.

Graham Steell's murmur

Because pressure in the pulmonary artery is normally quite low during diastole, significant regurgitation rarely occurs when the pulmonic

Understanding pulmonic insufficiency murmurs

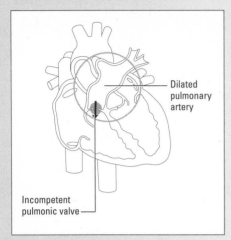

Dilated pulmonary artery

Incompetent pulmonic valve

Pulmonic insufficiency murmurs, including both Graham Steell's murmurs and normal pressure pulmonic valve murmurs, result when high-velocity blood flows backward from a dilated pulmonary artery across an incompetent pulmonic valve.

valve is functioning normally. However, if a patient has pulmonary hypertension, the pulmonary artery dilates. This, in turn, dilates the pulmonic valve ring, resulting in a relative pulmonic insufficiency. (See *Understanding pulmonic insufficiency murmurs.*) Graham Steell's murmur typically occurs only in severe pulmonary hypertension, when systolic pulmonary artery pressure exceeds 60 mm Hg. **(SOUND 40)**

Sound characteristics

The best place to hear a Graham Steell's murmur is along the left sternal border over the third and fourth intercostal spaces. The sound won't radiate to the right sternum. (See *Auscultating for pulmonic insufficiency murmurs.*)

Other characteristics include:
- murmur that may be present throughout diastole
- loud intensity, typically louder during inspiration
- variable duration
- high pitch, heard best with the diaphragm of the stethoscope
- blowing quality
- occurrence in early diastole
- a loud P_2 at the start, with a possible ejection sound
- location on an ECG after the end of the T wave
- decrescendo configuration. **(SOUND 40)**

Auscultating for pulmonic insufficiency murmurs

To hear either a Graham Steell's murmur or a normal pressure pulmonic valve murmur, listen along the left sternal border over the 3rd and 4th intercostal spaces, as shown here.

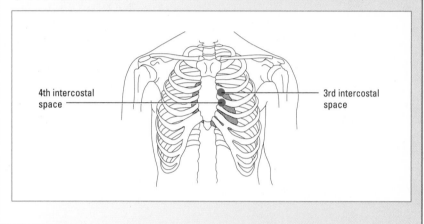

4th intercostal space

3rd intercostal space

Normal pressure pulmonic valve murmurs

Murmurs also may result from idiopathic pulmonary artery dilation or from congenital pulmonary valve insufficiency. In either case, the pulmonary artery diastolic pressure remains normal. Regurgitation occurs during isovolumic relaxation, after pressure in the right ventricle falls below pulmonary artery diastolic pressure. **(SOUND 41)**

Sound characteristics
You'll hear a normal pressure pulmonic valve murmur best along the left sternal border over the third and fourth intercostal spaces. The sound won't radiate to the right sternum.

> **KNOW-HOW** *Pulmonic insufficiency murmurs, particularly a normal pressure pulmonic valve murmur, intensify during inspiration.*
> *You'll hear the low-pressure regurgitant flow across the pulmonic valve as a brief crescendo-decrescendo, early diastolic murmur at the upper left sternal border. The sound becomes louder when the patient squats or takes a deep breath. The sound becomes softer when the patient exhales or performs Valsalva's maneuver. You may also note an S_3 or S_4 at the left mid-to-lower sternal border—a result of right ventricular hypertrophy or failure.*

Understanding mitral stenosis murmurs

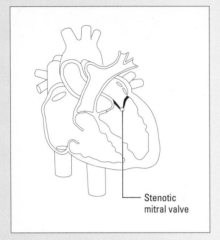

Mitral stenosis occurs when the mitral valve narrows or becomes obstructed, as shown here. The narrowed valve reduces forward blood flow from the left atrium to the left ventricle, causing a murmur.

Stenotic
mitral valve

Other characteristics include:
- occurrence in early diastole to middiastole
- typical start shortly after P_2
- rumbling quality, with a soft intensity and brief duration
- low pitch that's heard best with the bell of the stethoscope (unlike a Graham Steell's murmur)
- location on an ECG starting after the T wave and ending before the P wave
- crescendo-decrescendo configuration. **(SOUND 41)**

Mitral stenosis

Stenosis (narrowing) of the mitral valve usually results from chronic rheumatic heart disease caused by rheumatic fever. In rare instances, mitral stenosis may be congenital.

Chronic inflammation of the mitral valve leads to scarring and calcification. Consequently, the valve assumes a funnel shape and stops functioning normally. Rapid, turbulent blood flow through the narrowed, rigid valve produces the murmur characteristic of this condition. (See *Understanding mitral stenosis murmurs*.)

Mitral stenosis is sometimes associated with mitral regurgitation, so you may also hear a systolic murmur. If mitral stenosis has caused pul-

Auscultating for mitral stenosis murmurs

To best hear a mitral stenosis murmur, auscultate over the mitral area, as shown here, using the bell of the stethoscope.

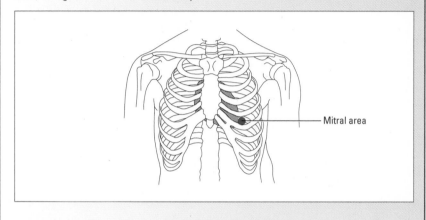

Mitral area

monary hypertension and right ventricular failure, tricuspid insufficiency may be the dominant murmur heard.

Sound characteristics

The best location for hearing a mitral stenosis murmur is near the apex of the heart, over the mitral area. (See *Auscultating for mitral stenosis murmurs.*)

 KNOW-HOW To enhance the sound of a mitral stenosis murmur, place the patient in a partial left lateral recumbent position. To further intensify the sound, have the patient perform maneuvers to increase cardiac output, such as raising his legs from a recumbent position, coughing several times, or performing some type of exercise for a few minutes.

Other characteristics include:
- variable intensity and duration
- low pitch, heard best with the bell of the stethoscope
- a rumbling quality that sounds like thunder
- occurrence shortly after S_2
- opening and closing snaps **(SOUND 42)**
- crescendo-decrescendo configuration. You'll particularly notice the presystolic crescendo—the result of increased turbulence before systole—in patients with a normal sinus rhythm. **(SOUND 43)**

Understanding tricuspid stenosis murmurs

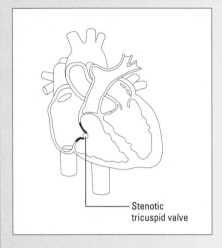

Stenotic
tricuspid valve

A tricuspid stenosis murmur results from a thickened and sclerotic tricuspid valve, as shown here, usually as a result of rheumatic fever.

The opening and closing snaps are an important diagnostic finding. The opening snap is a brief, loud sound produced when the stenotic valve suddenly halts its normal opening at the start of diastole. If the valve is calcified, S_1 is soft and the opening snap can't be heard. The murmur ends with a loud mitral component (M_1), or closing snap, which implies that the valve leaflets are mobile. The M_1 is usually palpable. **(SOUND 42)**

The more severe the stenosis, the longer the duration of the murmur. In severe mitral stenosis, the murmur is holodiastolic; in moderate stenosis, it appears in early and late diastole. On an ECG waveform, the murmur begins just after the T wave and ends during the QRS complex.

Tricuspid stenosis

In tricuspid stenosis, the tricuspid valves become thickened and sclerotic, obstructing blood flow from the right atrium to the right ventricle. This obstruction commonly causes the right heart to enlarge, which, in turn, may cause arrhythmias such as atrial fibrillation or flutter. Even if the patient has a normal sinus rhythm, you may notice

Auscultating for tricuspid stenosis murmurs

Unlike a mitral stenosis murmur—which is heard best over the apex of the heart—you'll hear a tricuspid stenosis murmur best when you listen over the tricuspid area at the left sternal border, as shown here.

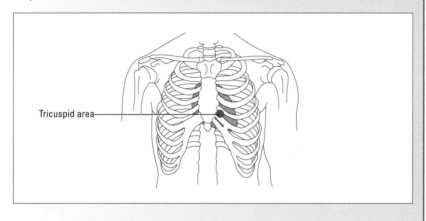

Tricuspid area

signs of atrial enlargement, such as tall P waves on inferior leads. (See *Understanding tricuspid stenosis murmurs.*)

Tricuspid stenosis rarely occurs alone. Typically caused by rheumatic fever, it usually occurs along with a mitral valve defect and, occasionally, aortic valve disease. On rare occasions, tricuspid stenosis may result from a congenital defect of the tricuspid valve.

Sound characteristics

You'll hear the murmur resulting from tricuspid stenosis best when auscultating over the tricuspid area while the patient is in a partial left lateral recumbent position. (See *Auscultating for tricuspid stenosis murmurs.*)

Other characteristics include:
- soft intensity that increases during inspiration and fades or disappears during expiration
- variable duration
- low pitch, heard best with the bell of the stethoscope
- a rumbling quality

- occurrence in middiastole to late diastole, starting shortly after a normal S_2 and ending just before S_1
- an opening snap that may precede the murmur, seldom audible but usually appearing on a phonocardiogram unless the snap is obscured by a mitral stenosis murmur **(SOUND 44)**
- location on an ECG starting just after the T wave and ending just before the QRS complex
- late diastolic crescendo or crescendo-decrescendo configuration in patients with normal sinus rhythm. **(SOUND 44)**

11 *Continuous murmurs*

Continuous murmurs begin in systole and persist without interruption throughout the cardiac cycle, late into diastole. These murmurs result from rapid blood flow through arteries or veins or from the shunting of blood. Shunting is caused by abnormal communication between the high-pressure arterial system and the low-pressure venous system.

Continuous murmurs may result from:
- cervical venous hum
- patent ductus arteriosus (PDA)
- mammary soufflé
- coarctation of the aorta or pulmonary artery
- aorticopulmonary window
- branch stenosis of the pulmonary artery
- systemic or pulmonic arteriovenous fistulas
- atrial fistulas.

Some of these produce a thrill, and many are associated with signs of right or left ventricular hypertrophy.

The three most common causes of continuous murmurs are:
- cervical venous hum
- PDA
- mammary soufflé.

Cervical venous hum

A cervical venous hum murmur—the most common continuous murmur—results when turbulent blood from the subclavian and internal jugular veins joins in the brachiocephalic vein before flowing down-

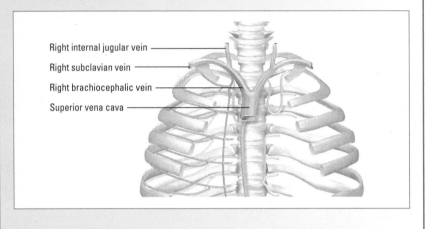

Understanding cervical venous hum murmurs

The subclavian and internal jugular veins join to form the brachiocephalic veins, which feed into the superior vena cava. A cervical venous hum murmur occurs when rapid blood flow from the subclavian and internal jugular veins meets in the brachiocephalic vein.

Right internal jugular vein

Right subclavian vein

Right brachiocephalic vein

Superior vena cava

ward into the superior vena cava. **(SOUND 45)** (See *Understanding cervical venous hum murmurs.*)

A normal, innocent occurrence in children, cervical venous hum murmurs are rare in adults. However, conditions causing hyperkinetic circulatory states, such as anemia, pregnancy, or thyrotoxicosis, may make the murmur more pronounced.

Sound characteristics

Although you may hear a cervical venous hum murmur on either side of the patient's neck, it's most audible on the right side. Have the patient sit with his head turned to the left while you auscultate the right side of his neck over the right supraclavicular fossa. Because the murmur has a low pitch, use the bell of the stethoscope while applying light pressure. (See *Auscultating for cervical venous hum murmurs.*)

Other characteristics include:

■ a soft quality

■ a faint intensity that increases during diastole, becoming louder between the second heart sound (S_2) and the first heart sound (S_1).

(SOUND 45)

Auscultating for cervical venous hum murmurs

To best hear a venous hum murmur, have the patient sit with his head turned to the left. Applying very light pressure, use the bell of the stethoscope to auscultate over the right supraclavicular fossa, just above the clavicle, as shown here.

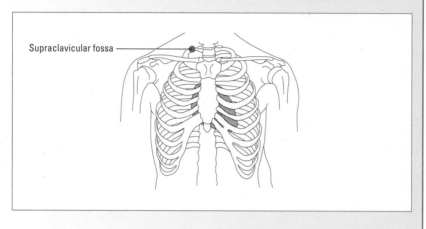

Supraclavicular fossa

- persistence throughout the cardiac cycle, with continuous timing (hence, the murmur's name)
- plateau shape in systole and crescendo-decrescendo configuration in diastole
- sometimes a sound loud enough to hear over the right sternal border, the sternum, or the left sternal border, which may be mistaken for a murmur caused by PDA, aortic stenosis, or aortic insufficiency
- disappearance of the hum when the patient performs Valsalva's maneuver, lies down, or turns his chin toward the stethoscope
- disappearance of the hum when you press on the jugular vein on the side you're auscultating, which you can do to differentiate between a venous hum and arterial or thyroid bruits, which don't disappear with pressure.

Patent ductus arteriosus

The ductus is a vascular channel between the aorta and the pulmonary artery. Open during fetal life, it normally closes shortly after birth. When the ductus remains open, as commonly occurs in premature in-

Understanding PDA murmurs

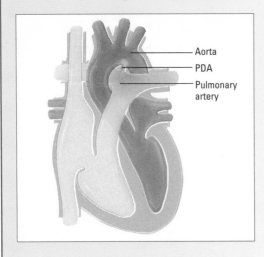

Aorta

PDA

Pulmonary artery

When the ductus remains open after birth, blood shunts from the aorta, an area of high pressure, to the pulmonary artery, an area of lower pressure. A patent ductus arteriosus (PDA) murmur results.

fants, blood shunts from the high-pressure aorta to the low-pressure pulmonary artery. (See *Understanding PDA murmurs.*)

Left untreated, a PDA may lead to irreversible pulmonary hypertension, which causes the shunt to reverse and flow from right to left. (This condition is known as Eisenmenger's syndrome.) A PDA usually presents as a systolic ejection murmur in newborns and develops into a continuous machinery murmur in older infants and children. **(SOUND 46)**

Sound characteristics

PDA murmurs are best heard when auscultating over the first and second intercostal spaces to the left of the sternum. The sound to this area is limited when the intensity is faint. If the murmur is loud, you may hear the systolic component along the left sternal border and, perhaps, over the mitral area as well. A loud PDA murmur may radiate to the patient's back, between his scapulae. A thrill may be palpable in loud PDA murmurs. (See *Auscultating for PDA murmurs.*)

Other characteristics include:
- a long duration, extending into diastole
- variable intensity, roughly correlating with ductus size, typically reaching maximum intensity late in systole and then fading during diastole

Auscultating for PDA murmurs

Patent ductus arteriosus (PDA) murmurs can be heard when auscultating over the 1st and 2nd intercostal spaces, as shown here. Unlike venous hums, murmurs from PDA sound louder to the left of the sternum. If the patient has a loud murmur, you may hear the systolic component along the left sternal border and, occasionally, over the mitral area, also shown here.

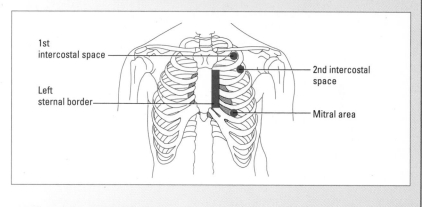

- possible increased intensity and duration with exercise
- continuous presence starting with or shortly after a normal S_1 and disappearing just before the next S_1
- difficulty hearing S_2 because the murmur peaks in late systole
- possible paradoxical split in S_2 if left ventricular ejection time is prolonged
- possible third heart sound (S_3) over the mitral area **(SOUND 46)**
- crescendo-decrescendo configuration (see *Differentiating between continuous murmurs,* page 146)
- pitch that varies with the pressure gradient between the aorta and the pulmonary artery across the PDA. Small PDA murmurs and those in newborns usually have a high pitch, heard equally well with the bell or the diaphragm of the stethoscope, and a rough, machinelike quality. As the PDA gets larger, or in older infants and children, the pitch may be medium to low.

*M*ammary souffle

Usually starting in the second or third trimester of pregnancy or during postpartum lactation, mammary souffle results from increased arterial

KNOW-HOW

Differentiating between continuous murmurs

When trying to distinguish a cervical venous hum murmur from one caused by patent ductus arteriosus (PDA), remember that a venous hum is:
- loudest above the clavicle
- usually heard best to the right of the sternum
- obliterated if you press on the jugular vein or place the patient in a supine position
- truly continuous
- usually louder during diastole.
   On the other hand, a PDA murmur is:
- heard best above the 1st and 2nd intercostal spaces over the left sternal border
- loudest during late systole and fading during diastole.

---

blood flow to the breast. The sound typically disappears at the second postpartum month or at the end of lactation. It also may occur in young adolescent girls because of increased blood flow to their developing breasts.

Sound characteristics

A mammary souffle is a systolic or continuous sound that's heard best over the second intercostal space at the midclavicular line (over one or both breasts) or over the left sternal border. Mammary souffle is best heard when the patient is lying down.

Other characteristics include:
- a soft blowing sound
- continuous or diamond shape
- systolic component starting after a slight delay following S_1
- disappearance of sound if the patient sits upright or stands, or if you apply firm pressure to the diaphragm of the stethoscope.

Keep in mind that the increased blood volume and cardiac output needed during pregnancy also may accentuate murmurs caused by stenotic heart valve lesions, such as mitral or aortic stenosis.

12 Other auscultatory sounds

In addition to the sounds already discussed, you may hear other sounds when performing a cardiac assessment. For example, if the patient has a prosthetic aortic or mitral valve, you'll hear sounds particular to the type of valve in use. In this chapter, we'll look at the sounds produced by prosthetic valves (aortic and mitral), pericardial friction rub, and mediastinal crunch. Becoming familiar with these sounds requires lots of practice. Be sure to take every opportunity to auscultate the hearts of patients who have prosthetic valves or those who have been diagnosed with valvular disease.

Understanding prosthetic valves

When a patient's heart valve malfunctions, usually because of stenosis or incompetence, he may receive a prosthetic valve. The most commonly replaced valves are the aortic and mitral valves. Tricuspid valves are occasionally replaced, but pulmonic valves rarely are.

When undergoing valve-replacement surgery, a patient may receive a mechanical valve or a valve made from biological tissue (bioprosthetic valve). The main types of mechanical valves include:
- bileaflet valve
- tilting-disk (single leaflet) valve
- ball-in-cage valve. (See *Types of prosthetic valves*, pages 148 to 150.)

Bioprosthetic valves may be made from animal tissue (heterograft or xenograft) or human tissue (homograft or allograft). Animal-tissue valves are made from the pericardium of pigs (porcine valves) or cows (bovine valves). Human tissue is rarely used.

(Text continues on page 151.)

Types of prosthetic valves

When a heart valve malfunctions, the patient may undergo surgery to replace it with a prosthetic valve. Here are the most commonly used valves.

Bileaflet valve

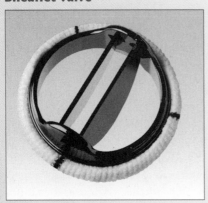

SJM Regent Valve.
Photo courtesy of St. Jude Medical.

Bovine valve

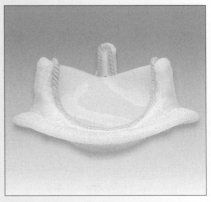

Carpentier-Edwards PERIMOUNT Pericardial
Bioprosthesis Valve.
Photo courtesy of Edwards Lifesciences.

The most commonly used valve type, a bileaflet valve consists of two semicircular leaflets that pivot on hinges. The leaflets swing open completely so that they lie parallel to the direction of blood flow. Because the leaflets don't completely close, some backflow occurs. However, this valve produces the type of central flow closest to that in a natural heart valve. In the United States, the St. Jude Medical valve is a commonly used bileaflet valve.

Bovine valves are constructed using bovine pericardial tissue. These valves provide a more symmetrical and complete opening for optimal hemodynamics. They also tend to be stronger and are more durable, and because they contain extra tissue, allow for future shrinkage. The Carpentier-Edwards PERIMOUNT valve is widely used.

Porcine valves

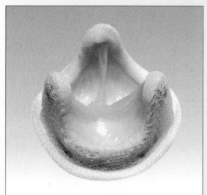

Hancock MO II Aortic Bioprosthesis.
Photo courtesy of Medtronic, Inc.

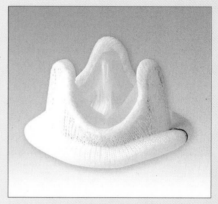

Carpentier-Edwards Duraflex Low Pressure
Bioprosthesis Valve.
Photo courtesy of Edwards Lifesciences.

Porcine valves consist of valve tissues from a pig that are sewn to a flexible or rigid frame called a *stent*. The stent is made from a metal alloy. Bent to form three U-shaped prongs, the stent is then covered with a Dacron cloth. Porcine valves include the Medtronic Hancock MO II Bioprosthesis valve and the Carpentier-Edwards Duraflex Low Pressure Bioprosthesis valve.

(continued)

Types of prosthetic valves *(continued)*

Tilting-disk valve

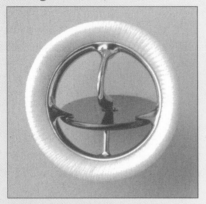

Medtronic Hall Mitral Valve.
Photo courtesy of Medtronic, Inc.

The tilting-disk valve was developed as an alternative to the ball-in-cage valve. This valve contains a flat, pivoting disk, mounted so that it floats between two hinges or struts. The valve closes when blood begins to flow backward and then reopens when the blood travels forward. The tilting-disk valve offers improved forward flow of blood while preventing backflow; it also causes minimal damage to blood cells. The most common tilting-disk valve is the Medtronic Hall valve.

Because the valve obstructs some blood flow, the hinges are strained. Over time, the hinges can break. This happened most with Björk-Shiley valves, which are no longer inserted, but you may still care for a patient who has such a valve.

Ball-in-cage valve

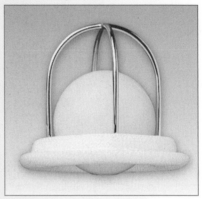

Starr-Edwards Silastic Ball Valve.
Photo courtesy of Edwards Lifesciences.

The ball-in-cage valve uses a small ball in a metal cage to keep blood flowing in a single direction. The first of its kind, this valve has several disadvantages. It's bulky and it causes the heart to work harder. Also, when blood cells collide with the valve they become damaged, causing them to release clotting factors, thereby increasing the patient's risk for thrombosis. Although this valve is no longer used, you may still see a patient who has one. The most commonly used ball-in-cage valve was the Starr-Edwards valve.

Mechanical valves are more durable and resist infection better than bioprosthetic valves. Because they last longer than bioprosthetic valves, a mechanical valve is usually the valve of choice for a younger patient. On the other hand, they're bulky and increase the risk of blood clotting. Therefore, patients with mechanical valves must take lifelong anticoagulant medication.

Bioprosthetic valves are a good alternative for some patients. These valves provide excellent hemodynamics, cause fewer problems than mechanical valves, and—because they're similar to human tissue—don't require lifelong anticoagulant medication. However, some of these valves are difficult to implant. They're also prone to calcification and, because they gradually deteriorate, they don't last as long as mechanical valves. (See *Pros and cons of mechanical and bioprosthetic valves,* page 152.)

AGE ALERT Because mechanical valves last a long time—sometimes a patient's lifetime—they're usually inserted in children and adults younger than age 40. However, these valves shouldn't be inserted in women of childbearing age. That's because pregnant women are at risk for developing blood clots. Also, patients with mechanical valves must always take an oral anticoagulant medication, and warfarin (an anticoagulant) may cause birth defects when given during the first trimester of pregnancy.

Bioprosthetic valves are also better suited for older patients. One reason is that calcification tends to occur on bioprosthetic valves, which can restrict blood flow or tear the valve leaflets. Patients younger than age 40 metabolize more calcium, placing them at a greater risk of developing calcification on a bioprosthetic valve. Further, bioprosthetic valves gradually degenerate and must be replaced, making them less desirable for a patient who wants to avoid future surgery. However, because patients with bioprosthetic valves don't need anticoagulant medication, these valves may be a suitable option for women of childbearing age or those who are pregnant.

Identifying prosthetic valve sounds and murmurs

Prosthetic valves produce characteristic sounds and murmurs. Some of the sounds you'll hear depend on the type of valve being auscultated, while other sounds occur regardless of valve type. For example, all prostheses, regardless of type or position, produce closing clicks and some also produce opening clicks. (The ball-in-cage valves and small porcine valves produce the loudest sounds.) However, an aortic prosthetic valve doesn't change a normal first heart sound (S_1), and a mitral prosthetic valve doesn't change a normal second heart sound (S_2).

Pros and cons of mechanical and bioprosthetic valves

Multiple factors influence the choice of which valve to use in which patient. This table lists the pros and cons of mechanical and bioprosthetic valves.

VALVE TYPE	PROS	CONS
Mechanical valve	▪ High durability ▪ Low risk of calcification ▪ Long function, possibly the patient's lifetime	▪ Increased risk of blood clots ▪ Need for lifelong anticoagulation therapy ▪ Damage to blood cells ▪ Poor hemodynamics ▪ Increased demand on the heart, which decreases cardiac efficiency
Bioprosthetic valve	▪ Superior hemodynamics ▪ No need for long-term anticoagulation therapy ▪ Protection of blood cells ▪ Fewer structural problems ▪ A design closer to that of a natural valve ▪ Conforms to surrounding body tissues	▪ Good durability, but not as good as mechanical valves ▪ Shorter lifespan (10 to 15 years), possibly requiring replacement ▪ Increased risk of calcification (particularly in children and adults younger than age 40)

During auscultation, if you notice that a previously heard prosthetic valve sound has disappeared or become muffled, or if you hear a new murmur, suspect prosthetic valve malfunction.

Aortic prosthetic valves

The surgeon places a prosthetic valve in the aortic orifice so that it opens during systole and closes at the beginning of diastole. Each type of valve—bileaflet valves, porcine and bovine valves, tilting-disk valves, and ball-in-cage valves—produces distinctive sounds and murmurs. **(SOUND 47)**

Nearly all aortic prosthetic valves obstruct outflow to some degree, which causes a soft early systolic or midsystolic ejection murmur. Regardless of valve type, auscultate over the aortic, tricuspid, and mitral areas to hear these sounds best. (See *Auscultating for aortic prosthetic valve murmurs.*)

Auscultating for aortic prosthetic valve murmurs

An aortic prosthetic valve typically produces a systolic ejection murmur that sounds like a mild murmur of aortic stenosis. You'll hear the sound best when auscultating over the aortic area, the tricuspid area along the left sternal border, and near the apex of the heart over the mitral area, as shown here.

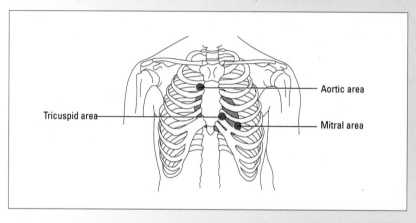

Aortic ball-in-cage valve

With a normally functioning aortic ball-in-cage valve, an aortic opening click follows and is louder than S_1. The sound is sharp and high-pitched, crisp in quality, and increasing in intensity with rising cardiac output. An aortic closing click replaces the aortic component (A_2).

Sound characteristics

Characteristics of a murmur generated by an aortic ball-in-cage valve typically include:
- loud intensity, making the murmur easy to hear
- medium pitch that's heard best with the diaphragm of the stethoscope
- midsystolic occurrence
- variable duration
- a crunchy, harsh quality
- no diastolic murmur (because ball-in-cage valves completely occlude outflow when closed)

- an interval between the aortic closing click and the pulmonic component (P_2) that's similar to the normal A_2–P_2 interval, normally widening during inspiration
- crescendo-decrescendo configuration.

Detecting a malfunctioning aortic ball-in-cage valve
Common findings with a malfunctioning aortic ball-in-cage valve include:
- soft or absent aortic opening click
- absent closing click.

You also may note a diastolic murmur and a prolonged systolic ejection murmur.

Aortic tilting-disk valve

With a normally functioning aortic tilting-disk valve, S_1 is unchanged.

Sound characteristics
You may hear an aortic opening click as well as a closing click, although the closing click won't be as loud as the closing click heard with a ball-in-cage valve. The interval between the aortic closing click and P_2 should be normal.

Other characteristics include:
- soft intensity (grade II/VI)
- short duration
- medium pitch that's heard best with the diaphragm of the stethoscope
- appearance during systole
- rough or harsh quality
- interval between the aortic closing click and P_2 that's similar to the normal A_2–P_2 interval, although it widens during inspiration
- crescendo-decrescendo configuration.

Detecting a malfunctioning aortic tilting-disk valve
If the patient has a malfunctioning aortic tilting-disk valve, you may discover some or all of these findings:
- absent aortic closing click
- diastolic murmur
- prolonged systolic ejection murmur.

Aortic bileaflet valve

A normally functioning aortic bileaflet valve produces a normal S_1.

Sound characteristics

You should note a loud, distinct closing click; you may also hear an opening click. Other characteristics include:

- soft intensity (grade II/VI)
- short duration
- medium pitch that's heard best with the diaphragm of the stethoscope
- appearance during systole
- rough or harsh quality
- interval between the aortic closing click and P_2 that's similar to the normal A_2–P_2 interval, widening during inspiration
- crescendo-decrescendo configuration.

Detecting a malfunctioning aortic bileaflet valve

If an aortic bileaflet valve malfunctions, you may notice an absent aortic closing click, a diastolic murmur, or both. You may also hear a prolonged systolic ejection murmur.

Aortic porcine and bovine valves

When auscultating a patient with an aortic porcine or bovine valve, you'll hear a normal S_2 with no opening click.

Sound characteristics

Characteristics of murmurs produced by aortic porcine and bovine valves include:

- soft intensity (grade II/VI)
- short duration
- medium pitch that's heard best with the diaphragm of the stethoscope
- rough or harsh quality
- no diastolic murmur (because these valves completely occlude the outflow of blood when closed)
- interval between the aortic closing sound and P_2 that's similar to the normal A_2–P_2 interval, widening during inspiration
- crescendo-decrescendo configuration.

Detecting a malfunctioning aortic porcine or bovine valve

If an aortic porcine or bovine valve malfunctions, you may hear a diastolic murmur or a prolonged systolic ejection murmur.

Auscultating for mitral prosthetic valve murmurs

A mitral prosthetic valve produces an early diastolic murmur. To hear this sound, auscultate over the mitral area near the heart's apex, as shown here.

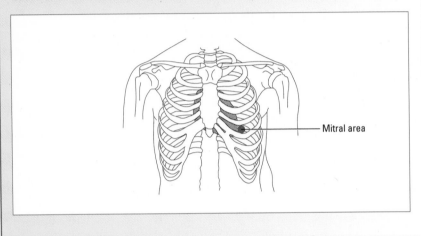

Mitral area

Mitral prosthetic valves

The surgeon places a prosthetic valve in the mitral orifice so it closes at the beginning of systole and opens during diastole. Mitral prosthetic valves produce distinctive sounds and murmurs. **(SOUND 48)** You'll hear the sounds best when auscultating over the mitral area, near the apex of the heart, with the patient in a partial left lateral recumbent position. (See *Auscultating for mitral prosthetic valve murmurs.*)

Mitral ball-in-cage valve

Normally functioning mitral ball-in-cage valves produce opening and closing clicks.

Sound characteristics
During auscultation, you'll notice a loud, high-frequency opening click after a normal S_2. You may also hear several clicks of varying intensity, which result from the bouncing of the ball in the cage. The closing click is less prominent than the opening click.

Auscultation may reveal:
- a short, soft (grade II/VI), rumbling diastolic murmur
- possible low-grade systolic murmur because the cage of this valve extends into the left ventricle and creates turbulent blood flow.

Detecting a malfunctioning mitral ball-in-cage valve

When a mitral ball-in-cage valve malfunctions in a patient with a normal sinus rhythm, you may discover that the sounds normally associated with the valve vary in intensity. Other signs of valve malfunction include:
- appearance of a short interval between A_2 and the mitral opening click (indicating high left atrial pressure)
- a holosystolic murmur (indicating mitral insufficiency)
- a change in the intensity and duration of the diastolic murmur (indicating mitral obstruction).

Mitral tilting-disk valve

A normally functioning mitral tilting-disk valve replaces the mitral component (M_1) with a mitral closing click.

Sound characteristics

The closing click produced by a mitral tilting-disk valve is distinct and high pitched. You may also hear:
- a mitral opening click after a normal S_2
- a short, soft, rumbling early diastolic murmur that sounds similar to a mitral stenosis murmur, except that it's brief and the presystolic component is absent.

Detecting a malfunctioning mitral tilting-disk valve

If a mitral tilting-disk valve malfunctions, you may notice that the mitral closing click has disappeared. Other possible findings include:
- a new diastolic murmur
- the intensification of a previously auscultated diastolic murmur
- a holosystolic mitral insufficiency murmur.

Mitral bileaflet valve

A mitral bileaflet valve produces a loud, high-pitched closing click that replaces M_1. Although rarely heard, a mitral opening click follows a normal S_2.

Sound characteristics

In addition to hearing a loud, high-pitched mitral closing click, you may also notice:

■ a short middiastolic rumble
■ a short, soft, rumbling early diastolic murmur that sounds similar to a mitral stenosis murmur (except that this murmur is brief and doesn't have a presystolic component).

Detecting a malfunctioning mitral bileaflet valve

If a mitral bileaflet valve malfunctions, it may produce a holosystolic murmur, a new diastolic murmur, or both.

Mitral porcine and bovine valves

Because bioprosthetic valves are made from tissue, they generate sounds similar to those of a natural heart valve.

Sound characteristics

You won't hear an opening sound, and the closing sound is similar to a normal M_1. You may hear a short, soft, rumbling early diastolic murmur that sounds similar to a mitral stenosis murmur. However, this murmur is brief and the presystolic component is absent.

Detecting a malfunctioning mitral porcine or bovine valve

A malfunctioning mitral porcine or bovine valve may produce a holosystolic mitral insufficiency murmur, a diastolic rumble associated with mitral stenosis, or both. It may also cause an early-to-midsystolic murmur after S_2 that's followed by an opening sound.

Identifying other abnormal sounds

Other abnormal sounds you may identify during auscultation include a pericardial friction rub and a mediastinal crunch.

Pericardial friction rub

When inflamed pericardial surfaces rub together, they produce a characteristic high-pitched friction noise known as *pericardial friction rub.*
(SOUND 49)

A classic sign of pericardial inflammation (pericarditis), a pericardial friction rub may result from a viral or bacterial infection, radiation

KNOW-HOW

Tips for hearing pericardial friction rubs

If you suspect that your patient has a pericardial friction rub, first have him lean forward to bring the heart closer to the chest wall. Alternatively, place him in a knee-chest position. Then, using the diaphragm of the stethoscope, auscultate initially over Erb's point. Listen intently as the patient exhales slowly and force-fully. Remain alert for high-pitched, leathery, scratchy sounds whenever the patient's heart contracts.

A friction rub may consist of between one and three components, which you'll hear during atrial systole, ventricular systole, or ventricular diastole. As a result, the sounds produced by the rub may coincide with the first or second heart sound.

Persist or cease?

To differentiate a pericardial friction rub from a pleural friction rub, have the pa-tient hold his breath. The sound from a pericardial friction rub persists, while the sound from a pleural friction rub ceases.

---

therapy to the chest, or cardiac trauma. Pericardial friction rubs com-monly occur in patients who have had pericardiotomies. You also may hear one for a few hours or a few days following a myocardial infarc-tion.

Sound characteristics

In addition to being audible, a pericardial friction rub also may be pal-pable in the tricuspid and xiphoid areas. (See *tips for hearing pericar-dial friction rubs.* Also see *Auscultating for pericardial friction rubs,* page 160.) Characteristics of pericardial friction rub include:
- high pitch (heard best with the diaphragm of the stethoscope)
- grating or scratchy quality
- loudness, possibly growing even louder during inspiration.

During each cardiac cycle, you may hear a pericardial friction rub during systole as well as during early and late diastole. **(SOUND 49)** The diastolic component may last for only a few hours.

Auscultating for pericardial friction rubs

To best hear a pericardial friction rub, auscultate over the tricuspid and xiphoid areas, as shown here.

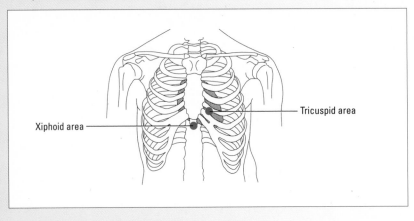

Auscultating for mediastinal crunch

Remember that with mediastinal crunch, the sound is synchronized with the patient's heartbeat, not with his respirations. To auscultate this sound, place the patient in a left lateral decubitus position and listen over the left sternal border, as shown here.

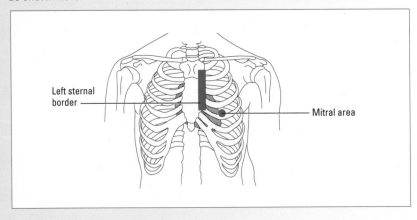

Mediastinal crunch

If air enters the mediastinum (such as in a pneumomediastinum), movements of the heart displace the air, producing a crunchy or crackling sound known as mediastinal crunch. Also called *Hamman's sign,* the sounds may occur randomly or in a consistent pattern. **(SOUND 50)** Patients with mediastinal crunch commonly have sub-cutaneous emphysema (air trapped beneath the skin). As with stridor, treat mediastinal crunch as a medical emergency.

Sound characteristics

To hear the noises produced by mediastinal crunch, place the patient in a left lateral decubitus position and then auscultate along the left sternal border. (See *Auscultating for mediastinal crunch.*) You'll notice that the noises, which should have a crunching or scratching quality, are synchronous with the heartbeat. **(SOUND 50)**

13 Cardiovascular disorders

Despite advances in detection and treatment, cardiovascular disease remains the leading cause of death in the United States. Myocardial infarction (MI) is the number one cause of cardiovascular-related deaths. If your patient is diagnosed with a cardiovascular disorder, you'll need to understand the disease process, what causes it, and what to look for. Each disease may produce distinctive heart sounds. The more you listen to heart sounds, the more you'll feel comfortable and confident about understanding what you're hearing.

Abdominal aortic aneurysm

An abnormal dilation or ballooning in the arterial wall, abdominal aortic aneurysm most commonly occurs in the aorta between the renal arteries and iliac branches. More than half of patients with untreated abdominal aneurysms die within 2 years of diagnosis, mainly from rupture of the aneurysm. More than 85% die within 5 years.

Causes

Aneurysms commonly result from atherosclerosis, which weakens the aortic wall and gradually distends the lumen. Other causes include:
- fungal infection (mycotic aneurysm) of the aortic arch and descending segments
- congenital disorders, such as coarctation of the aorta and Marfan syndrome (a multisystemic connective tissue disorder characterized by such skeletal changes as abnormally long limbs, cardiovascular defects that commonly include dilation of the ascending aorta, and other deformities)

162

■ trauma
■ syphilis
■ hypertension (in dissecting aneurysm).

Pathophysiology

Degenerative changes in the muscular layer of the aorta (tunica media) create a focal weakness, allowing the inner layer (tunica intima) and outer layer (tunica adventitia) to stretch outward. The resulting outward bulge is called an *aneurysm.* Blood pressure in the aorta progressively weakens the vessel walls and enlarges the aneurysm.

Assessment

Auscultation of the abdomen will reveal a blowing murmur over the aorta or a whooshing sound (bruit). Other signs and symptoms may include:
■ an asymptomatic pulsating mass in the periumbilical area
■ abdominal tenderness on deep palpation
■ lumbar pain that radiates to the flank and groin (a sign of imminent rupture).
   If the aneurysm ruptures, look for:
■ severe, persistent abdominal and back pain, mimicking renal or ureteral colic
■ weakness
■ sweating
■ tachycardia
■ hypotension.

Cardiac tamponade

In cardiac tamponade, a rapid rise in intrapericardial pressure equalizes right and left ventricular diastolic pressures, impairing diastolic filling of the heart. The rise in pressure usually results from blood or fluid accumulation in the pericardial sac.
   The fibrous wall of the pericardial sac can stretch to accommodate up to 2 L of fluid. If fluid accumulates slowly, as in pericardial effusion caused by cancer, signs and symptoms may not be evident immediately. However, as little as 200 ml of fluid can create an emergency if it accumulates rapidly. Left untreated, cardiogenic shock and death can occur.

CASE CLIP

Responding to cardiac tamponade

Mrs. M., a 72-year-old white woman was recovering well on the postoperative open heart unit after uncomplicated cardiovascular surgery to replace her diseased mitral valve. Throughout the day, Mrs. M. experienced an increase in shortness of breath, which she attributed to an increase in her activity. Around dinnertime, Mrs. M. called her nurse. On examination, Mrs. M. described the increasing shortness of breath and said that now it even happens at rest. Mrs. M. had a pulse oximeter reading of 90% and physical examination revealed tachypneic and labored breathing. Her vital signs were:

- temperature: 98.9° F (31.2° C)
- heart rate (HR): 103 beats/minute
- respiratory rate: 30 breaths/minute
- blood pressure (BP): 84/30 mm Hg.

Mrs. M. was alert and oriented and sitting up in bed with moderate distress. On auscultation, her lungs were found to be clear. There was prominent jugular vein distention noted. On assessment, her heart sounds were muffled and distant. Concerned that Mrs. M. was deteriorating, the nurse summoned the rapid response team (RRT). Mrs. M.'s nurse described the situation to the RRT as a postoperative open heart patient experiencing hypotension and increasing dyspnea. The RRT further assessed Mrs. M. Based on the cardiac surgery history, hypotension, weak pulses, and findings of muffled and distant heart sounds, the RRT considered cardiac tamponade as the most likely cause of Mrs. M.'s signs and symptoms.

Stat echocardiogram, electrocardiogram (ECG), and chest X-ray were ordered. The cardiovascular surgical team was also notified. An additional I.V. line was secured and I.V. fluids started. Mrs. M.'s ECG showed sinus tachycardia with low voltage, which is recognized as smaller than normal QRS complexes. The echocardiogram validated the diagnosis of a pericardial effusion and tamponade.

Throughout the ongoing assessment, Mrs. M.'s vital signs remained unchanged:

- HR: 100 to 120 beats/minute
- BP: 88/60 mm Hg.

The nurse verified that a current type and crossmatch was available and requested that 2 units of packed RBCs be held. Labs were sent, including a CBC, PT, PTT, and INR. The RRT remained with the patient until the cardiovascular surgeon was available. The RRT discussed with Mrs. M. and her nurse that if there was any further deterioration in her condition they would perform an emergency pericardiocentesis at the bedside but would work on keeping her stable until the procedure could be performed in the operating room.

Cardiac tamponade is a life-threatening condition and a medical emergency. A short time later, Mrs. M. was transported to the cardiovascular operating room and the effusion was drained through pericardiocentesis by her cardiovascular surgeon.

Causes

Cardiac tamponade may result from:
- effusion caused by cancer, bacterial infection, tuberculosis and, rarely, acute rheumatic fever
- hemorrhage caused by trauma, cardiac surgery, or perforation during cardiac or central venous catheterization (see *Responding to cardiac tamponade*)
- hemorrhage from nontraumatic causes, such as rupture of the heart or great vessels or anticoagulant therapy in a patient with pericarditis
- pericarditis
- acute MI
- chronic renal failure during dialysis
- an adverse reaction from procainamide, hydralazine, minoxidil, isoniazid, penicillin, or daunorubicin
- connective tissue disorders, such as rheumatoid arthritis, systemic lupus erythematosus, rheumatic fever, vasculitis, or scleroderma.

When cardiac tamponade has no known cause, it's called *Dressler's syndrome.*

Pathophysiology

In cardiac tamponade, the progressive accumulation of fluid in the pericardium compresses the heart chambers. This obstructs blood flow into the ventricles and reduces the amount of blood that can be pumped out of the heart with each contraction.

Every time the ventricles contract, more fluid accumulates in the pericardial sac. This further limits the amount of blood that can fill the chamber during the next cardiac cycle. Reduced cardiac output may be fatal without prompt treatment.

Assessment

Cardiac tamponade has three classic features, which are known as *Beck's triad:*
- elevated central venous pressure with jugular vein distention
- muffled heart sounds
- pulsus paradoxus (inspiratory drop in systemic blood pressure greater than 10 mm Hg).

Unfortunately, Beck's triad is an extremely late finding. Pericardial friction rubs also aren't reliable indicators of tamponade; they're typically absent with large effusions.

Other signs and symptoms include:
- orthopnea
- diaphoresis

- anxiety
- restlessness
- cyanosis
- weak, rapid peripheral pulse.

Cardiogenic shock

Sometimes called *pump failure*, cardiogenic shock is a condition of diminished cardiac output that severely impairs tissue perfusion. It reflects severe left-sided heart failure and occurs as a serious complication in some patients hospitalized with acute MI.

Cardiogenic shock typically affects patients whose area of infarction exceeds 40% of the heart's muscle mass. In such patients, the fatality rate may exceed 85%. Most patients with cardiogenic shock die within 24 hours of onset. The prognosis for those who survive is extremely poor.

Causes

Most cases of cardiogenic shock result from acute myocardial ischemia. Other related causes include:
- toxicity to drugs such as doxorubicin
- infectious or inflammatory processes such as acute myocarditis
- certain drugs, such as beta-adrenergic blockers and calcium channel blockers
- mechanical causes, such as valvular dysfunction, tamponade, or cardiomyopathy.

Patients with preexisting myocardial damage, arrhythmias, or diabetes are at increased risk for developing cardiogenic shock.

Pathophysiology

As cardiac output falls, aortic and carotid baroreceptors prompt sympathetic nervous system responses, which increase heart rate, left ventricular filling pressure, and peripheral resistance to flow, to enhance venous return to the heart.

These compensatory responses initially stabilize the patient but later cause his condition to deteriorate as the oxygen demands of his already compromised heart rise. These events compose a vicious cycle of low cardiac output, sympathetic compensation, myocardial ischemia, and even lower cardiac output.

Assessment

The first step is to try to discover the cause of cardiogenic shock. For example, careful examination may reveal a mechanical cause, such as papillary rupture, valve dysfunction, myocardial wall or septal rupture, cardiac tamponade, or aortic aneurysm. These conditions usually respond well to surgical intervention.

If you detect a loud murmur, suspect valve dysfunction as the cause of the condition. Muffled heart tones along with jugular vein distention and pulsus paradoxus suggest tamponade.

Cardiogenic shock produces signs of poor tissue perfusion, such as:
- cold, pale, clammy skin
- drop in systolic blood pressure to 30 mm Hg below the baseline, or a sustained reading below 80 mm Hg that isn't attributable to medication
- tachycardia
- rapid, shallow respirations
- oliguria (urine output less than 20 ml/hour)
- restlessness
- confusion
- narrowing pulse pressure
- cyanosis
- gallop rhythm and faint heart sounds.

Dilated cardiomyopathy

Dilated cardiomyopathy occurs when myocardial muscle fibers sustain extensive damage. Disturbances in myocardial metabolism and gross dilation of the heart's chambers cause the heart to assume a globular shape. Dilated cardiomyopathy leads to intractable heart failure, arrhythmias, and emboli. Usually not diagnosed until its advanced stages, this disorder carries a poor prognosis.

Causes

The primary cause of dilated cardiomyopathy is unknown. Although the relationship remains unclear, it occasionally occurs secondary to:
- viral or bacterial infections
- hypertension
- peripartum syndrome (related to toxemia)
- ischemic heart disease or valve disease
- drug hypersensitivity or chemotherapy
- cardiotoxic effects of drugs or alcohol
- pregnancy

- anemia
- thyrotoxicosis.

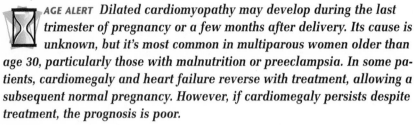 *AGE ALERT Dilated cardiomyopathy may develop during the last trimester of pregnancy or a few months after delivery. Its cause is unknown, but it's most common in multiparous women older than age 30, particularly those with malnutrition or preeclampsia. In some patients, cardiomegaly and heart failure reverse with treatment, allowing a subsequent normal pregnancy. However, if cardiomegaly persists despite treatment, the prognosis is poor.*

Pathophysiology

Dilated cardiomyopathy is characterized by both a grossly dilated, weak ventricle that contracts poorly as well as, to a lesser degree, myocardial hypertrophy. Increased volumes and pressures cause all four heart chambers to dilate. This leads to blood pooling, thrombus formation, and possible embolization.

If hypertrophy coexists, the heart ejects blood less efficiently. A large volume of blood remains in the left ventricle after systole, leading to heart failure.

Assessment

The patient may develop:
- shortness of breath (orthopnea, exertional dyspnea, or paroxysmal nocturnal dyspnea)
- fatigue
- dry cough at night
- edema
- liver engorgement
- jugular vein distention
- peripheral cyanosis
- sinus tachycardia
- atrial fibrillation
- diffuse apical impulses
- pansystolic murmur (as a result of mitral and tricuspid insufficiency secondary to cardiomegaly and weak papillary muscles)
- third heart sound (S_3) and fourth heart sound (S_4) gallop rhythms.

Endocarditis

Endocarditis (infection of the endocardium, heart valves, or cardiac prosthesis) results from bacterial or fungal invasion. Untreated endocarditis usually proves fatal but, with proper treatment, 70% of patients recover. Prognosis becomes much worse when endocarditis causes severe valve damage, leading to insufficiency and heart failure, or when it involves a prosthetic valve.

Causes

Causative organisms include:
- group A nonhemolytic *streptococci*
- *Pneumococcus*
- *Staphylococcus*
- *Enterococcus*
- rarely, *gonococcus.*

Most cases of endocarditis occur in patients who abuse I.V. drugs. Also at high risk are those who have prosthetic heart valves, a previous history of endocarditis (even in the absence of other heart disease), complex cyanotic congenital heart disease, or surgically constructed systemic pulmonary shunts or conduits. If endocarditis does occur in these patients, it's more likely to be severe and have a poor prognosis.

Patients with a moderate risk of severe infection include those who have an uncorrected patent ductus arteriosus, ventricular septal defect, primum atrial septal defect, coarctation of the aorta, or a bicuspid aortic valve. Patients who have valve dysfunction from rheumatic heart disease or collagen vascular disease as well as those with hypertrophic cardiomyopathy also have a moderate risk of developing endocarditis.

Pathophysiology

Infection triggers the accumulation of fibrin and platelets on valve tissue. Friable, wartlike, vegetative growths form on the heart valves, the endocardial lining of a heart chamber, or the endothelium of a blood vessel. These growths may cover valve surfaces, causing ulceration and necrosis, and may also extend to the chordae tendineae. Ultimately, the growths may embolize to the spleen, kidneys, central nervous system, and lungs. (See *Effects of endocarditis,* page 170.)

Assessment

Early clinical features are usually nonspecific and include:
- weakness
- fatigue
- weight loss
- anorexia
- arthralgia

Effects of endocarditis

This illustration shows vegetative growths on the endocardium produced by fibrin and platelet deposits on infection sites.

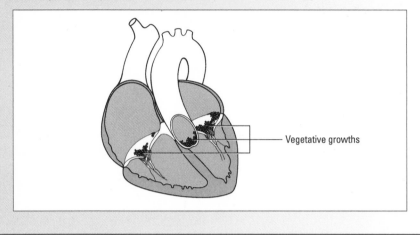

Vegetative growths

■ night sweats

■ intermittent fever (which may recur for weeks)

■ loud, regurgitant murmur (typical of underlying rheumatic or congenital heart disease)

■ murmur that changes or appears suddenly, accompanied by fever.

*H*eart failure

When the myocardium can't pump effectively enough to meet the body's metabolic needs, heart failure results. Pump failure usually occurs in a damaged left ventricle but may also happen in a right ventricle. Usually, left-sided heart failure develops first. Heart failure is classified as:

■ acute or chronic

■ left-sided or right-sided (see *Understanding left- and right-sided heart failure*)

■ systolic or diastolic.

Symptoms of heart failure may severely restrict a patient's ability to perform activities of daily living. While advances in diagnosis and

(Text continues on page 174.)

Understanding left- and right-sided heart failure

These illustrations show how myocardial damage leads to heart failure.

Left-sided heart failure

1. Increased workload and end-diastolic volume enlarge the left ventricle (as shown below). Lack of oxygen causes the ventricle to enlarge with stretched tissue rather than functional tissue. The patient may have an increased heart rate, pale and cool skin, tingling in the limbs, decreased cardiac output, and arrhythmias.

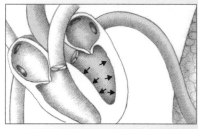

2. Diminished left ventricular function allows blood to pool in the ventricle and the atrium and eventually back up into the pulmonary veins and capillaries (as shown below). At this stage, the patient may have dyspnea on exertion, confusion, dizziness, orthostatic hypotension, decreased peripheral pulses and pulse pressure, cyanosis, and an S_3 gallop.

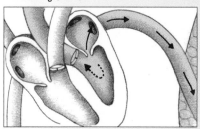

3. As pulmonary circulation becomes engorged, rising capillary pressure pushes sodium (Na) and water (H_2O) into the interstitial space (as shown below), causing pulmonary edema. You'll note coughing, subclavian retractions, crackles, tachypnea, elevated pulmonary artery pressure, diminished pulmonary compliance, and increased partial pressure of carbon dioxide.

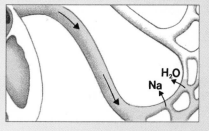

(continued)

Understanding left- and right-sided heart failure *(continued)*

4. When the patient lies down, fluid in the limbs moves into the systemic circulation. Because the left ventricle can't handle the increased venous return, fluid pools in the pulmonary circulation, worsening pulmonary edema (as shown below). You may note decreased breath sounds, dullness on percussion, crackles, and orthopnea.

5. The right ventricle may now become stressed because it's pumping against greater pulmonary vascular resistance and left ventricular pressure (as shown below). When this occurs, the patient's symptoms worsen.

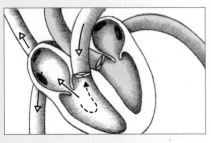

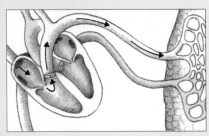

Right-sided heart failure

1. The stressed right ventricle enlarges with the formation of stretched tissue (as shown below). Increasing conduction time and deviation of the heart from its normal axis can cause arrhythmias. If the patient doesn't already have left-sided heart failure, he may develop an increased heart rate, cool skin, cyanosis, decreased cardiac output, palpitations, and dyspnea.

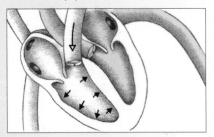

2. Blood pools in the right ventricle and right atrium. The backed-up blood causes pressure and congestion in the vena cava and systemic circulation (as shown below). The patient will have elevated central venous pressure, jugular vein distention, and hepatojugular reflux.

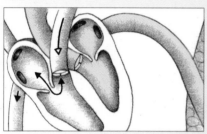

3. Backed-up blood also distends the visceral veins, especially the hepatic vein. As the liver and spleen become engorged (as shown below), their function is impaired. The patient may develop anorexia, nausea, abdominal pain, palpable liver and spleen, weakness, and dyspnea secondary to abdominal distention.

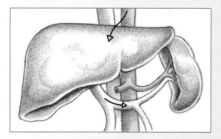

4. Rising capillary pressure forces excess fluid from the capillaries into the interstitial space (as shown below). This causes tissue edema, especially in the lower extremities and abdomen. The patient may have weight gain, pitting edema, and nocturia.

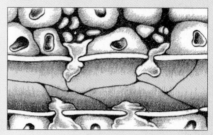

treatment have greatly improved the outcome for many patients, the prognosis still depends on the underlying cause and its response to treatment.

Causes

Many cardiovascular disorders can lead to heart failure, including:
- arrhythmias
- atherosclerotic heart disease
- cardiomyopathy
- congenital heart disease
- hypertension
- ischemic heart disease
- MI
- rheumatic heart disease
- valve diseases.

Noncardiovascular causes of heart failure include:
- acute blood loss
- chronic obstructive pulmonary disease
- increased environmental temperature or humidity
- pregnancy and childbirth
- pulmonary embolism
- severe infection
- severe physical or mental stress
- thyrotoxicosis.

Pathophysiology

The patient's underlying condition determines whether heart failure is acute or chronic. Typically, systolic or diastolic overload combined with myocardial weakness leads to heart failure.

As stress on the heart muscle reaches a critical level, the heart's ability to contract declines and cardiac output falls. At the same time, venous blood flow to the heart remains the same, which causes the ventricles to fill with increased volumes of blood.

As cardiac output falls, the body responds by:
- increasing sympathetic activity
- releasing renin from the kidneys
- triggering anaerobic metabolism in affected cells
- inciting peripheral cells to extract more oxygen.

The heart also tries to compensate. For example, as the end-diastolic fiber length increases, the ventricular muscle dilates and increases the force of contractions. Called the *Frank-Starling curve,* this is a short-term compensation measure. A long-term measure occurs as the ventricle hypertrophies. An enlarged ventricle allows the heart to contract more forcefully, ejecting more blood into circulation.

Assessment

Clinical signs of left-sided heart failure include:
- dyspnea (initially upon exertion)
- paroxysmal nocturnal dyspnea
- Cheyne-Stokes respirations
- cough
- orthopnea
- tachycardia
- fatigue
- muscle weakness
- edema and weight gain
- irritability
- restlessness
- shortened attention span
- S_3 or S_4 heart sounds
- bibasilar crackles.

A patient with right-sided heart failure may develop:
- edema (initially dependent)
- jugular vein distention
- hepatomegaly.

Hypertrophic cardiomyopathy

A primary disease of the cardiac muscle, hypertrophic cardiomyopathy is characterized by disproportionate, asymmetrical thickening of the interventricular septum, particularly the anterior-superior portion. It affects both diastolic and systolic function.

The thickened septum obstructs blood flow through the aortic valve. As the papillary muscles become affected, mitral insufficiency occurs. The course of the disease varies; some patients progressively deteriorate, while others remain stable for several years. Sudden cardiac death can occur.

Causes

Almost all patients inherit hypertrophic cardiomyopathy as a non–sex-linked autosomal dominant trait.

Pathophysiology

In hypertrophic cardiomyopathy, the left ventricular muscle enlarges, becoming stiff and noncompliant. Too little room remains in the ventricle to receive an adequate volume of blood during diastole, which reduces cardiac output. The heart compensates by increasing the rate and force of contractions. As left ventricular volume diminishes and filling pressure rises, pulmonary venous pressure also rises, leading to venous congestion and dyspnea.

Assessment

On auscultation, you may hear an S_3 or S_4 as well as a systolic ejection murmur. Heard best along the left sternal border at the apex of the heart, the murmur may have a medium pitch and is commonly intensified by Valsalva's maneuver.

Other clinical features include:
- angina pectoris
- arrhythmias
- dyspnea
- syncope
- heart failure
- pulsus biferiens
- irregular pulse (with atrial fibrillation).

Myocardial infarction

Characterized as an acute coronary syndrome, MI is an occlusion of a coronary artery that leads to oxygen deprivation, myocardial ischemia, and eventual necrosis. The extent of functional impairment and the patient's prognosis depend on the size and location of the infarct, the condition of the uninvolved myocardium, the potential for collateral circulation, and the effectiveness of compensatory mechanisms. In the United States, MI is the leading cause of death in adults.

Causes

MI can arise from any condition in which myocardial oxygen supply can't keep pace with demand, including:
- coronary artery disease
- coronary artery emboli
- thrombus
- coronary artery spasm
- severe hematologic and coagulation disorders
- myocardial contusion
- congenital coronary artery anomalies.

Certain risk factors increase a patient's vulnerability to MI. These factors include a family history of MI; gender (men are more susceptible); hypertension; smoking; elevated serum triglyceride, cholesterol, and low-density lipoprotein levels; diabetes mellitus; obesity; sedentary lifestyle; aging; stress; and menopause.

Pathophysiology

MI results from prolonged ischemia to the myocardium with irreversible cell damage and muscle death. Functionally, MI causes:
- reduced contractility with abnormal wall motion
- altered left ventricular compliance
- reduced stroke volume
- reduced ejection fraction
- elevated left ventricular end-diastolic pressures.

Assessment

MI causes severe, persistent chest pain that's unrelieved by rest or nitroglycerin. The patient may describe the pain as crushing or squeezing. Usually substernal, pain may radiate to the left arm, jaw, neck, or shoulder blades. Other signs and symptoms include a feeling of impending doom, fatigue, nausea and vomiting, shortness of breath, cool extremities, perspiration, anxiety, hypotension or hypertension, palpable precordial pulse and, possibly, muffled heart sounds. Women are less likely to experience chest pain with an MI, but may complain of pain in the shoulder blades, jaw, and upper back. Women also complain of fatigue, palpitations, and indigestion.

AGE ALERT *Elderly patients are more prone to complications and death after an acute MI. The most common complications include:*
- *arrhythmias*
- *cardiogenic shock*
- *heart failure resulting in pulmonary edema*
- *pericarditis.*

Other complications include:
- *rupture of the atrial or ventricular septum, ventricular wall, or valves*
- *ventricular aneurysms*
- *mural thrombi, leading to cerebral or pulmonary emboli*
- *extension of the original infarction*
- *post-MI pericarditis, called* Dressler's syndrome *(occurring days to weeks after an MI, causing residual pain, malaise, and fever)*
- *psychological problems because of fear of another MI or as a result of an organic brain disorder from tissue hypoxia*
- *personality changes.*

Pericarditis

Pericarditis is acute or chronic inflammation of the pericardium, the fibroserous sac that envelops, supports, and protects the heart. Acute pericarditis can be fibrinous or effusive, with purulent serous or hemorrhagic exudate. Chronic constrictive pericarditis characteristically leads to dense fibrous pericardial thickening.

Because pericarditis commonly coexists with other conditions, diagnosis of acute pericarditis depends on typical clinical features and the elimination of other possible causes. Prognosis depends on the underlying cause. Most patients recover from acute pericarditis, unless constriction occurs.

Causes

Pericarditis may result from:
- bacterial, fungal, or viral infection (infectious pericarditis)
- neoplasm (primary or metastatic from lungs, breasts, or other organs)
- high-dose radiation to the chest
- uremia

■ hypersensitivity or autoimmune diseases, such as rheumatic fever (the most common cause of pericarditis in children), systemic lupus erythematosus, and rheumatoid arthritis
■ postcardiac injury, such as MI (which later causes an autoimmune reaction [Dressler's syndrome] in the pericardium), trauma, and surgery that leaves the pericardium intact but causes blood to leak into the pericardial cavity
■ drugs, such as hydralazine and procainamide
■ idiopathic factors (most common in acute pericarditis)
■ aortic aneurysm with pericardial leakage and myxedema with cholesterol deposits in the pericardium (less commonly).

Pathophysiology

Inflammation causes the pericardium to become thickened and fibrotic. If it doesn't heal completely after an acute episode, it may slowly calcify, forming a firm scar around the heart. This scarring interferes with diastolic filling of the ventricles.

Assessment

Auscultation may reveal a pericardial friction rub. A classic sign, this grating sound occurs as the heart moves. (See *Responding to pericarditis*, page 180.) To hear a friction rub best, firmly apply the diaphragm of your stethoscope to the patient's left lower sternal border. Listen as the patient forcefully exhales while leaning forward or while he's on his hands and knees in bed.

This rub occurs in three phases corresponding with atrial systole, ventricular systole, and ventricular diastole. However, it's uncommon for all three phases to be heard clinically. Occasionally, friction rub is heard only briefly or not at all.

Other signs and symptoms of pericarditis include:
■ sharp, sudden pain that usually starts over the sternum and radiates to the neck, shoulders, back, and arms (unlike the pain of MI, pericardial pain is usually pleuritic, increasing with deep inspiration and decreasing when the patient sits up and leans forward)
■ signs similar to those of chronic right-sided heart failure, such as fluid retention, ascites, and hepatomegaly (with chronic constrictive pericarditis).

CASE CLIP

Responding to pericarditis

Mr. G. was a 45-year-old white male with a history of poorly controlled hypertension, and nonischemic cardiomyopathy induced by his long history of sustained alcoholism despite medical advice to stop drinking. He presented to his practitioner's office for evaluation of increased shortness of breath, edema, and some mild chest discomfort. Associated symptoms included malaise and a low-grade fever. Before the onset of his symptoms he had suffered from flulike symptoms of fever and aches and pains with no associated cold symptoms such as a cough. After a physical examination, the practitioner admitted Mr. G. to the hospital for exacerbation of heart failure and ordered I.V. diuretics, positive inotropes, and angiotensin-converting enzyme inhibitors.

On the second day of admission, Mr. G. complained to his nurse that he was experiencing anxiety and an increase in his chest discomfort, now describing it as a sharp, persistent chest pain that became worse with deep inspiration or position changes. On assessment, his vital signs were:
- temperature: 99.7° F (37.6° C)
- heart rate (HR): 101 beats/minute and regular
- respiratory rate (RR): 20 breaths/minute and unlabored
- blood pressure (BP): 165/90 mm Hg.

His breath sounds were clear and his abdomen was flat, soft, nontender and with normal bowel sounds time in all four quadrants. There was no jugular vein distention and no peripheral edema. The nurse administered I.V. midazolam, per orders, to treat what was assessed as alcohol withdrawal symptoms. Over the next 2 hours, Mr. G.'s anxiety continued to increase and he continued to complain about chest pain. Reassessment of his vital signs were unchanged from earlier.

Before administering a second dose of midazolam, the rapid response team (RRT) was activated. Assessment by the RRT found an anxious male, with these vital signs:
- HR: 122 beats/minute
- RR: 32 breaths/per minute
- BP: 170/92 mm Hg
- pulse oximetry: 98%.

The RRT administered sublingual nitroglycerin; Mr. G. described no relief of the chest pain with the nitroglycerin. Further physical assessment and a review of the patient's history, including electrocardiogram (ECG), revealed a heart sound with a harsh grating S_1 and S_2 recognized as a pericardial friction rub. The ECG showed global ST-wave elevation. Because of Mr. G.'s anxiety and the severity of his symptoms, a stat echocardiogram was also completed and interpreted as not significant findings for pericardial tamponade.

Based on the history, physical assessment revealing a pericardial friction rub, and an ECG showing global ST-wave elevation, the RRT concluded that Mr. G. had pericarditis. Mr. G.'s practitioner was notified of the findings and started Mr. G. on anti-inflammatory medications and analgesics for the pain.

Restrictive cardiomyopathy

Characterized by restricted ventricular filling and failure to contract completely during systole, restrictive cardiomyopathy is a rare disorder of the myocardial musculature that results in low cardiac output and eventually endocardial fibrosis and thickening. If severe, it's irreversible.

Causes

The cause of primary restrictive cardiomyopathy remains unknown. In amyloidosis, infiltration of amyloid into the intracellular spaces in the myocardium, endocardium, and subendocardium may lead to restrictive cardiomyopathy syndrome.

Pathophysiology

Left ventricular hypertrophy and endocardial fibrosis limit myocardial contraction and emptying during systole as well as ventricular relaxation and filling during diastole. As a result, cardiac output falls.

Assessment

Auscultation may reveal lung crackles, abnormal or distant heart sounds, and S_3 or S_4 gallop rhythms. Other findings include:
- fatigue
- dyspnea
- orthopnea
- chest pain
- generalized edema
- liver engorgement
- peripheral cyanosis
- pallor.

Rheumatic fever and rheumatic heart disease

A systemic inflammatory disease of childhood, acute rheumatic fever develops after infection of the upper respiratory tract with group A beta-hemolytic streptococci. Commonly recurrent, rheumatic fever mainly involves the heart, joints, central nervous system, skin, and subcutaneous tissues. If rheumatic fever isn't treated, scarring and deformity of cardiac structures result in rheumatic heart disease.

Worldwide, 15 to 20 million new cases of rheumatic fever are reported each year. The disease strikes most often during the cool, damp weather of winter and early spring. In the United States, it's most common in northern climates.

Causes

Apparently, a hypersensitivity reaction to a group A beta-hemolytic streptococcal infection causes rheumatic fever. Because only about 3% of people infected with *Streptococcus* contract rheumatic fever, altered immune response probably influences its development or recurrence.

Because rheumatic fever tends to run in families, patients may be genetically predisposed to the disease. Environmental factors also seem to play a role. For example, in lower socioeconomic groups, the illness typically occurs in children between ages 5 and 15, probably because of malnutrition and crowded living conditions.

Pathophysiology

Inflammation of the heart (carditis) develops in up to half of patients with rheumatic fever and may affect the endocardium, myocardium, or pericardium during the early acute phase. The extent of heart damage depends on where the infection strikes.

Myocarditis produces characteristic lesions called *Aschoff's bodies* in the interstitial tissue of the heart and also causes cells in the interstitial collagen to swell and fragment. This leads to the formation of progressively fibrotic nodules and interstitial scars.

Endocarditis causes valve leaflets to swell and erode. Vegetative deposits also form on affected valves. Endocarditis typically strikes the mitral valve in females and the aortic valve in males. It may affect the tricuspid valve in either gender but rarely affects the pulmonic valve. Long-term effects include destruction of the mitral and aortic valves, which may lead to pericardial effusion and fatal heart failure. Of the patients who survive this complication, about 20% die within 10 years.

Pancarditis is the most serious and second most common complication of rheumatic fever. In advanced cases, patients may complain of dyspnea, mild to moderate chest discomfort, pleuritic chest pain, edema, cough, or orthopnea.

Assessment

In 95% of patients, rheumatic fever follows a streptococcal infection within a few days to 6 weeks and causes a temperature of at least 100.4° F (38° C). Most patients complain of migratory joint pain or polyarthritis. Swelling, redness, and signs of effusion—usually in the knees, ankles, elbows, and hips—also occur.

The most common sign of cardiac involvement is a new murmur (usually the result of valve insufficiency) and tachycardia out of proportion to fever. Other cardiac manifestations include heart failure and pericarditis.

Part two

Breath sounds

14 Respiratory anatomy and physiology

The respiratory system consists of the upper respiratory tract, lower respiratory tract (including the lungs), and thoracic cavity. In addition to maintaining the exchange of oxygen and carbon dioxide in the lungs and tissues, the respiratory system also helps regulate the body's acid-base balance.

Upper respiratory tract

The upper respiratory tract consists mainly of the:
- mouth
- nose
- pharynx
- nasopharynx
- oropharynx
- laryngopharynx
- larynx.

These structures warm and humidify inspired air. They're also responsible for taste, smell, and the chewing and swallowing of food. (See *The respiratory system*.)

Nose and nasal passages

Air enters the body through the nares (nostrils). In the nares, small hairs known as *vibrissae* filter out dust and large foreign particles. Air then passes into the two nasal passages, which are separated by the septum. Cartilage forms the anterior walls of the nasal passages; bony structures (known as turbinates, or conchae) form the posterior walls.

The respiratory system

Use this illustration to help yourself visualize the structures of the respiratory system.

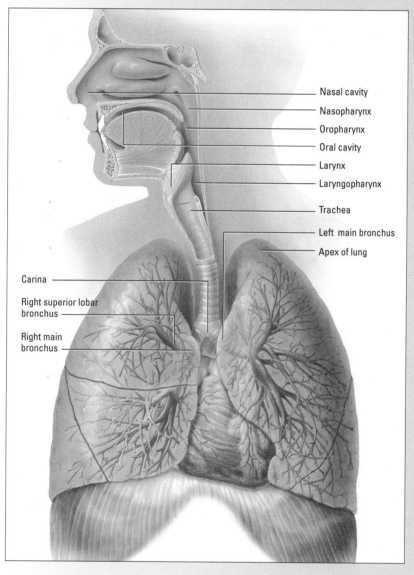

Nasal cavity

Nasopharynx

Oropharynx

Oral cavity

Larynx

Laryngopharynx

Trachea

Left main bronchus

Apex of lung

Carina

Right superior lobar bronchus

Right main bronchus

The superior, middle, and inferior turbinates are separated by grooves, called meatus.

The curved bony turbinates and their mucosal covering ease breathing by warming, filtering, and humidifying inhaled air before it passes into the nasopharynx. Their mucus layer also traps finer foreign particles, which the cilia carry to the pharynx to be swallowed.

The sinuses serve as resonators for sound production and provide mucus. Four pairs of paranasal sinuses open into the internal nose:

- The maxillary sinuses are located on the cheeks below the eyes.
- The frontal sinuses are located above the eyebrows.
- The ethmoidal and sphenoidal sinuses are located behind the eyes and nose in the head.

Pharynx and nasopharynx

The pharynx is composed of striated muscle and lined with a mucous membrane. It serves as a passageway for air entering from the nose. Air passes from the nasal cavity into the muscular nasopharynx through the choanae, a pair of posterior openings in the nasal cavity that remain constantly open.

Oropharynx and laryngopharynx

The oropharynx is the posterior wall of the mouth. It connects the nasopharynx and the laryngopharynx. The laryngopharynx extends to the esophagus and larynx.

Larynx

The larynx connects the pharynx to the trachea, and it contains the vocal cords. Muscles and cartilage form the walls of the larynx, including the large, shield-shaped thyroid cartilage situated under the jaw line.

 AGE ALERT In children, the larynx and glottis are positioned higher in the neck, creating a greater risk for aspiration.

Lower respiratory tract

The lower respiratory tract consists of the trachea, bronchi, and lungs. Functionally, the lower tract is subdivided into the conducting airways and the acinus. The acinus serves as the area of gas exchange. A mucous membrane that contains hairlike cilia lines the lower tract. Cilia constantly clean the tract and carry foreign matter upward for swallowing or expectoration.

Conducting airways

The conducting airways, which contain the trachea and bronchi, help facilitate gas exchange.

Trachea

The trachea extends from the cricoid cartilage at the top to the carina (also called the tracheal bifurcation). The carina is a ridge-shaped structure at the level of the sixth or seventh thoracic vertebra. The adult trachea is about 1″ (2.5 cm) in diameter and 4″ (10 cm) long to the bifurcation. C-shaped cartilage rings reinforce and protect the trachea to prevent it from collapsing.

 *AGE ALERT **In children, the trachea is shorter with a more acute angle at the bifurcation of the right bronchus. The smaller diameter of the trachea results in increased airway resistance.***

Bronchi

The primary bronchi begin at the carina. The left mainstem bronchus delivers air to the left lung. The right mainstem bronchus—shorter, wider, and more vertical than the left—supplies air to the right lung.

The mainstem bronchi divide into five lobar bronchi (secondary bronchi). Along with blood vessels, nerves, and lymphatics, the secondary bronchi enter the pleural cavities and the lungs at the hilum. Located behind the heart, the hilum is a slit on the lung's medial surface where the lungs are anchored.

Each lobar bronchus enters a lobe in each lung. In its lobe, each of the lobar bronchi branches into segmental bronchi (tertiary bronchi). The segments continue to branch into smaller and smaller bronchi, finally branching into bronchioles.

The larger bronchi consist of cartilage, smooth muscle, and epithelium. As the bronchi become smaller, they first lose cartilage, then smooth muscle until, finally, the smallest bronchioles consist of just a single layer of epithelial cells.

Acinus

Each bronchiole includes an acinus—the chief respiratory unit for gas exchange. The acinus consists of respiratory bronchioles and alveoli. (See *The pulmonary airway,* page 190.)

The pulmonary airway

As shown in this illustration, each bronchiole contains terminal bronchioles and the acinus, consisting of respiratory bronchioles and alveolar sacs.

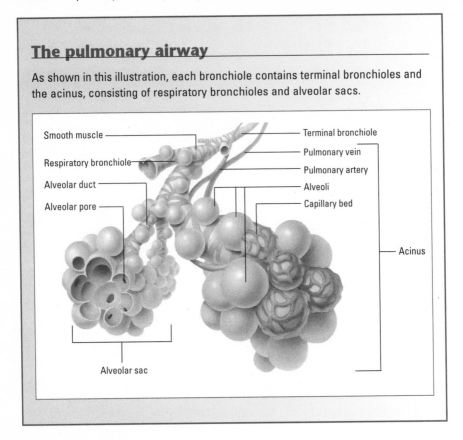

Smooth muscle

Respiratory bronchiole

Alveolar duct

Alveolar pore

Terminal bronchiole

Pulmonary vein

Pulmonary artery

Alveoli

Capillary bed

Acinus

Alveolar sac

Respiratory bronchioles

In the acinus, terminal bronchioles branch into yet smaller respiratory bronchioles. The respiratory bronchioles feed directly into alveoli at sites along their walls.

Alveolar walls contain two basic epithelial cell types:
- Type I cells, which are the most abundant, are thin, flat, squamous cells. Gas exchange occurs across these cells.
- Type II cells secrete surfactant, a substance that coats the alveolus and promotes gas exchange by lowering surface tension.

Alveoli

The respiratory bronchioles eventually become alveolar ducts, which terminate in clusters of capillary-swathed alveoli called alveolar sacs. Gas exchange takes place through the alveoli.

AGE ALERT *Adults have about 10 times the number of alveoli as infants, who have alveoli that are larger with less elastic recoil. The number of alveoli reaches that of an adult by age 12.*

Lungs and accessory structures

The cone-shaped lungs hang suspended in the right and left pleural cavities, straddling the heart and anchored by root and pulmonary ligaments.

The right lung is shorter, broader, and larger than the left. It has three lobes and handles 55% of gas exchange. The left lung has two lobes. Each lung's concave base rests on the diaphragm; the apex extends about ½" (1.3 cm) above the first rib.

Pleura and pleural cavities

The pleura—the serous membrane that totally encloses the lung—is composed of a visceral layer and a parietal layer. The visceral pleura hugs the entire lung surface, including the areas between the lobes. The parietal pleura lines the inner surface of the chest wall and upper surface of the diaphragm.

The pleural cavity—the tiny area between the visceral and parietal pleural layers—contains a thin film of serous fluid. This fluid has two functions:
- It lubricates the pleural surfaces so that they slide smoothly against each other as the lungs expand and contract.
- It creates a bond between the layers that causes the lungs to move with the chest wall during breathing.

Thoracic cavity

The thoracic cavity is an area that's surrounded by the:
- diaphragm (below)
- the scalene muscles and fasciae of the neck (above)
- ribs
- intercostal muscles
- vertebrae
- sternum
- ligaments (around the circumference).

In the thoracic cavity are the mediastinum and the thoracic cage.

Mediastinum

The space between the lungs is called the mediastinum. It contains the:

- heart and pericardium
- thoracic aorta
- pulmonary artery and veins
- venae cavae and azygos veins
- thymus, lymph nodes, and vessels
- trachea, esophagus, and thoracic duct
- vagus, cardiac, and phrenic nerves.

Thoracic cage

Composed of bone and cartilage, the thoracic cage supports and protects the lungs, allowing them to expand and contract. The thoracic cage is divided into a posterior and an anterior portion.

Posterior thoracic cage

The vertebral column and 12 pairs of ribs comprise the posterior portion of the thoracic cage. The ribs constitute the major portion of the thoracic cage. They extend from the thoracic vertebrae toward the anterior thorax.

Anterior thoracic cage

The anterior thoracic cage consists of the:

- manubrium
- sternum
- xiphoid process
- ribs.

It protects the mediastinal organs that lie between the right and left pleural cavities.

Ribs 1 through 7 attach directly to the sternum; ribs 8 through 10 attach to the cartilage of the preceding rib. The other two pairs of ribs are free-floating. In other words, they don't attach to any part of the anterior thoracic cage. Rib 11 ends anterolaterally, and rib 12 ends laterally.

The lower portion of the rib cage (costal margins) near the xiphoid process forms the borders of the costal angle—an angle of about 90 degrees in a normal person. (See *Locating lung structures in the thoracic cage.*)

Locating lung structures in the thoracic cage

The ribs, vertebrae, and other structures of the thoracic cage act as landmarks that you can use to identify underlying structures, as illustrated here.

From the front

■ The base of each lung rests at the level of the 6th rib at the midclavicular line and the 8th rib at the midaxillary line.

■ The apex of each lung extends about ¾" to 1½" (2 to 4 cm) above the inner aspects of the clavicles.

■ The upper lobe of the right lung ends level with the 4th rib at the midclavicular line and with the 5th rib at the midaxillary line.

■ The middle lobe of the right lung extends triangularly from the 4th to the 6th rib at the midclavicular line and to the 5th rib at the midaxillary line.

■ Because the left lung doesn't have a middle lobe, the upper lobe of the left lung ends level with the 4th rib at the midclavicular line and with the 5th rib at the midaxillary line.

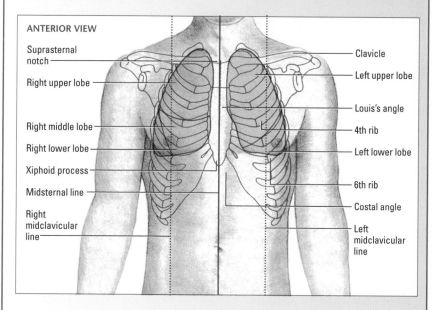

(continued)

Locating lung structures in the thoracic cage *(continued)*

From the back
- The lungs extend from the cervical area to the level of the 10th thoracic vertebra (T10). On deep inspiration, the lungs may descend to T12.
- An imaginary line from T3 level along the inferior border of the scapulae to the 5th rib at the midaxillary line separates the upper lobes of both lungs.
- The upper lobes lie above T3; the lower lobes lie below T3 and extend to the level of T10.
- The diaphragm originates around the 9th or 10th rib.

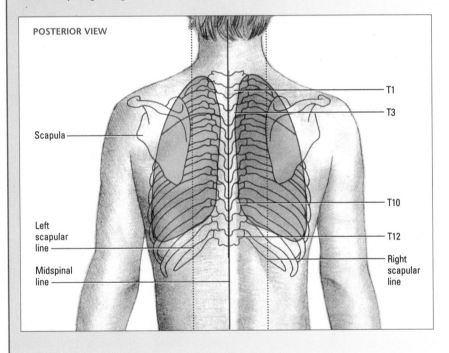

POSTERIOR VIEW

T1
T3
Scapula
T10
Left scapular line
T12
Right scapular line
Midspinal line

Above the anterior thorax is a depression called the suprasternal notch. Because the rib cage doesn't cover the suprasternal notch, as it does the rest of the thorax, the trachea and aortic pulsation can be palpated here.

From the side

■ The right and left lateral rib cage covers the lobes of the right and left lungs, respectively.

■ Beneath these structures, the lungs extend from just above the clavicles to the level of the 8th rib.

■ The left lateral thorax allows access to two lobes; the right lateral thorax, to three lobes.

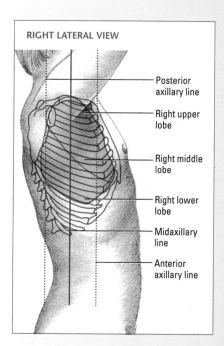

RIGHT LATERAL VIEW

Posterior axillary line

Right upper lobe

Right middle lobe

Right lower lobe

Midaxillary line

Anterior axillary line

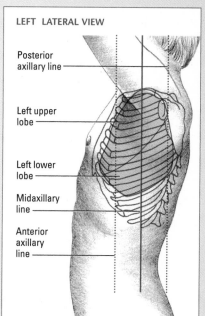

LEFT LATERAL VIEW

Posterior axillary line

Left upper lobe

Left lower lobe

Midaxillary line

Anterior axillary line

Inspiration and expiration

Breathing involves two actions: inspiration (an active process) and expiration (a relatively passive process). Both actions rely on respiratory muscle function and the effects of pressure differences in the lungs.

Mechanics of respiration

The muscles of respiration help the chest cavity expand and contract. Pressure differences between atmospheric air and the lungs help produce air movement. These illustrations show the muscles that work together to allow inspiration and expiration.

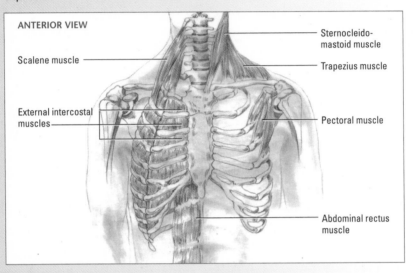

ANTERIOR VIEW

Scalene muscle

External intercostal muscles

Sternocleido-mastoid muscle

Trapezius muscle

Pectoral muscle

Abdominal rectus muscle

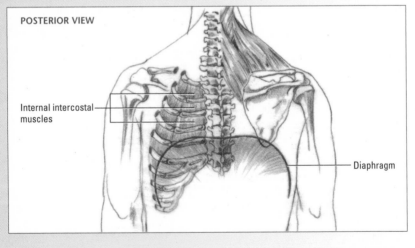

POSTERIOR VIEW

Internal intercostal muscles

Diaphragm

During normal respiration, the external intercostal muscles aid the diaphragm, the major muscle of respiration. The diaphragm descends to lengthen the chest cavity, while the external intercostal muscles (located between and along the lower borders of the ribs) contract to expand the anteroposterior diameter. This coordinated action causes inspiration. Rising of the diaphragm and relaxation of the intercostal muscles cause expiration. (See *Mechanics of respiration.*)

 AGE ALERT **Children are diaphragmatic breathers until about age 6 because of their poorly developed intercostal muscles.**

Forced inspiration and active expiration

During exercise, when the body needs increased oxygenation, or in certain disease states that require forced inspiration and active expiration, the accessory muscles of respiration also participate.

Forced inspiration

During forced inspiration:
- the pectoral muscles (upper chest) raise the chest to increase the anteroposterior diameter
- the sternocleidomastoid muscles (side of neck) raise the sternum
- the scalene muscles (in the neck) elevate, fix, and expand the upper chest
- the posterior trapezius muscles (upper back) raise the thoracic cage.

Active expiration

During active expiration, the internal intercostal muscles contract to shorten the chest's transverse diameter, and the abdominal rectus muscles pull down the lower chest, thus depressing the lower ribs.

Oxygen-depleted blood enters the lungs from the pulmonary artery of the heart's right ventricle. It then flows through the main pulmonary arteries into the smaller vessels of the pleural cavities and the main bronchi, through the arterioles and, eventually, to the capillary networks in the alveoli. In the alveoli, gas exchange—oxygen and carbon dioxide diffusion—takes place. (See *Tracing pulmonary circulation,* page 198.)

Tracing pulmonary circulation

The right and left pulmonary arteries carry deoxygenated blood from the right side of the heart to the lungs. These arteries divide into distal branches, called *arterioles,* that eventually terminate as a concentrated capillary network in the alveoli and alveolar sacs, where gas exchange occurs.

Venules—the end branches of the pulmonary veins—collect oxygenated blood from the capillaries and transport it to larger vessels, which in turn lead to the pulmonary veins. These veins enter the left side of the heart and provide oxygenated blood to the body.

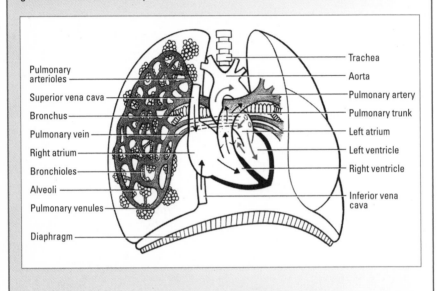

Labels (left): Pulmonary arterioles · Superior vena cava · Bronchus · Pulmonary vein · Right atrium · Bronchioles · Alveoli · Pulmonary venules · Diaphragm

Labels (right): Trachea · Aorta · Pulmonary artery · Pulmonary trunk · Left atrium · Left ventricle · Right ventricle · Inferior vena cava

External and internal respiration

Effective respiration consists of gas exchange in the lungs, called external respiration, and gas exchange in the tissues, called internal respiration.

External respiration occurs through three processes:
- *ventilation*—gas distribution into and out of the pulmonary airways
- *pulmonary perfusion*—blood flow from the right side of the heart, through the pulmonary circulation, and into the left side of the heart
- *diffusion*—gas movement through a semipermeable membrane from an area of greater concentration to one of lesser concentration.

Internal respiration occurs only through diffusion.

Ventilation

Ventilation is the distribution of gases (oxygen and carbon dioxide) into and out of the pulmonary airways. Problems within the nervous, musculoskeletal, and pulmonary systems greatly compromise breathing effectiveness.

Involuntary breathing results from stimulation of the respiratory center in the medulla and the pons of the brain. The medulla controls the rate and depth of respiration; the pons moderates the rhythm of the switch from inspiration to expiration.

The medulla controls ventilation primarily by stimulating contraction of the diaphragm and external intercostal muscles. Because the adult thorax is flexible, contraction of the chest muscles changes its shape. In turn, this produces intrapulmonary pressure changes, triggering inspiration.

Many factors affect airflow distribution. These factors include:
- airflow pattern (see, *Comparing airflow patterns,* page 228)
- volume and location of the functional reserve capacity (air retained in the alveoli that prevents their collapse during respiration)
- degree of intrapulmonary resistance
- presence of lung disease.

If airflow is disrupted for any reason, airflow distribution follows the path of least resistance.

Other musculoskeletal and intrapulmonary factors can affect airflow and, in turn, may affect breathing. For example, forced breathing, as in emphysema, activates accessory muscles of respiration. Using these muscles increases the workload of breathing, which requires additional oxygen and results in less-efficient ventilation.

Other airflow alterations can also increase oxygen and energy demand and cause respiratory muscle fatigue. These conditions include interference with expansion of the lungs or thorax (changes in compliance) and interference with airflow in the tracheobronchial tree (changes in resistance).

AGE ALERT *Aging causes decreased compliance of the lungs and chest wall. In the older adult, airway closure and a loss of surface area results in decreased ventilation at the bases of the lungs. Although maximal lung function decreases with age, breathing should remain adequate. In nonsmokers, changes caused by aging don't cause clinically significant airway obstruction or dyspnea.*

What happens in ventilation-perfusion mismatch

Ideally, the amount of air in the alveoli (a reflection of ventilation) should match the amount of blood in the capillaries (a reflection of perfusion). This allows gas exchange to proceed smoothly.

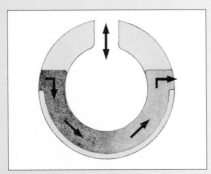

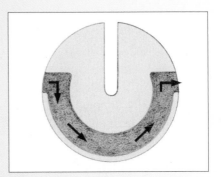

Normal

In the normal lung, ventilation closely matches perfusion.

Shunt

Perfusion without ventilation usually results from airway obstruction, particularly that caused by acute diseases, such as atelectasis and pneumonia.

Pulmonary perfusion

Pulmonary perfusion refers to blood flow from the right side of the heart, through the pulmonary circulation, and into the left side of the heart. Perfusion aids external respiration. Normal pulmonary blood flow allows alveolar gas exchange; however, many factors may interfere with gas transport to the alveoli. Here are some examples:

■ Cardiac output less than the average of 5 L/minute reduces blood flow, which decreases gas exchange.

■ Elevations in pulmonary and systemic resistance also reduce blood flow.

■ Abnormal or insufficient hemoglobin picks up less oxygen for exchange.

Gravity can affect oxygen and carbon dioxide transport in a positive way. Gravity causes more unoxygenated blood to travel to the lower

In actuality, the ventilation-perfusion ($\dot{V}/\dot{Q}$) ratio is unequal: The alveoli receive air at a rate of about 4 L/minute, while the capillaries supply blood at a rate of about 5 L/minute. This creates a $\dot{V}/\dot{Q}$ mismatch of 4:5, or 0.8.

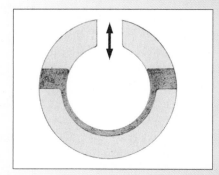

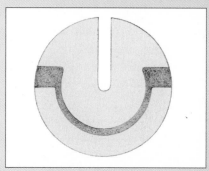

Dead-space ventilation
Normal ventilation without perfusion usually results from a perfusion defect, such as pulmonary embolism.

Silent unit
Absence of ventilation and perfusion usually stems from multiple causes, such as pulmonary embolism with resultant acute respiratory distress syndrome and emphysema.

and middle lung lobes than to the upper lobes. This explains why ventilation and perfusion differ in various parts of the lungs. Areas where perfusion and ventilation are similar have what's referred to as a ventilation-perfusion match; in such areas, gas exchange is most efficient. (See *What happens in ventilation-perfusion mismatch.*)

Diffusion

In diffusion, oxygen and carbon dioxide molecules move between the alveoli and capillaries. The movement always proceeds from an area of greater concentration to one of lesser concentration. In the process, oxygen moves across the alveolar and capillary membranes, dissolves in the plasma, and then passes through the red blood cell (RBC) membrane. Carbon dioxide moves in the opposite direction.

For successful diffusion, the epithelial membranes lining the alveoli and capillaries must be intact. Both the alveolar epithelium and the capillary endothelium are composed of a single layer of cells. Between these layers are tiny interstitial spaces filled with elastin and collagen.

Normally, oxygen and carbon dioxide move easily through all of these layers. Oxygen moves from the alveoli into the bloodstream. Once there, most of it binds with hemoglobin to form oxyhemoglobin; however, a small portion dissolves in plasma. (The portion of oxygen that dissolves in plasma can be measured as the partial pressure of oxygen in arterial blood, or PaO_2.) When oxygen binds with hemoglobin, it displaces carbon dioxide (the by-product of metabolism). The carbon dioxide diffuses from the RBCs into the blood, where it travels to the alveoli.

After oxygen binds to hemoglobin, the RBCs travel to the tissues. Through cellular diffusion, the RBCs release oxygen and absorb carbon dioxide. The RBCs then transport the carbon dioxide back to the lungs for removal during expiration. This is known as internal respiration. (See *Exchanging gases.*)

Acid-base balance

Oxygen taken up in the lungs is transported to the tissues by the circulatory system, which exchanges it for carbon dioxide produced by metabolism in body cells. Because carbon dioxide is more soluble than oxygen, it dissolves in the blood. In the blood, most of the carbon dioxide forms bicarbonate (base) and smaller amounts form carbonic acid (acid).

The lungs control bicarbonate levels by converting bicarbonate to carbon dioxide and water for excretion. In response to signals from the medulla, the lungs can change the rate and depth of breathing. This change allows for adjustments in the amount of carbon dioxide loss, which help to maintain acid-base balance.

For example, in metabolic acidosis (a condition resulting from excess acid retention or excess bicarbonate loss), the lungs increase the rate and depth of ventilation to eliminate excess carbon dioxide, thus reducing carbonic acid levels. In metabolic alkalosis (a condition resulting from excess bicarbonate retention), the rate and depth of ventilation decrease so that carbon dioxide can be retained; this increases carbonic acid levels.

When the lungs don't function properly, an acid-base imbalance results. For example, they can cause respiratory acidosis through hypo-

Exchanging gases

Gas exchange occurs very rapidly in the millions of tiny, thin-membraned alveoli in the respiratory units. Inside these air sacs, oxygen from inhaled air diffuses into the blood while carbon dioxide diffuses from the blood into the air and is exhaled. Blood then circulates throughout the body, delivering oxygen and picking up carbon dioxide. Finally, the blood returns to the lungs to be oxygenated again.

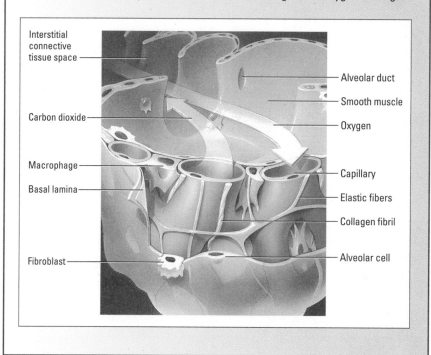

ventilation (reduced rate and depth of ventilation), which leads to carbon dioxide retention. They can also cause respiratory alkalosis through hyperventilation (increased rate and depth of ventilation), which leads to carbon dioxide elimination.

15 *Respiratory assessment*

Because the respiratory system is critical to survival, respiratory assessment is a critical nursing responsibility. Performing a comprehensive respiratory assessment requires knowledge of the respiratory system, accurate data collection, and recognition of abnormalities. A detailed health history and systematic physical examination can help you identify patients' respiratory changes.

Obtaining a health history

The information you gain from the patient's medical history helps you understand his present symptoms. When obtaining a health history, focus your questioning on complaints of shortness of breath, cough, sputum production, wheezing, and chest pain. (See *Respiratory facts.*)

Begin by asking the patient about any complaints of dyspnea (shortness of breath). Ask him to rate his usual level of dyspnea on a scale of 0 to 10, in which 0 means no dyspnea and 10 means the worst he has experienced. Then ask him to rate the level that day.

Next, ask the patient to grade his dyspnea as it relates to activity. (See *Grading dyspnea,* page 206.) In addition, you might also ask these questions:

■ What do you do to relieve the dyspnea?
■ How well does it work?

A patient with orthopnea (shortness of breath when lying down) tends to sleep with his upper body elevated. Ask this patient how many pillows he uses. The answer describes the severity of orthopnea. For example, a patient who uses three pillows can be said to have "three-pillow orthopnea."

KNOW-HOW

Respiratory facts

A quick review of your patient's health history can reveal a lot about his current problem.

Coughing

Coughing clears unwanted material from the tracheobronchial tree. Also, sputum from the bronchial tubes traps foreign matter and protects the lungs from damage.

Pain sites

The lungs don't contain pain receptors; however, chest pain may be caused by inflammation of the pleura or the costochondral joints at the midclavicular line or at the edge of the sternum.

How much oxygen?

Patients with chronically high partial pressure of arterial carbon dioxide ($PaCO_2$), such as those with chronic obstructive pulmonary disease or a neuromuscular disease, may be stimulated to breathe by a low oxygen level (the hypoxic drive) rather than by a slightly high $PaCO_2$ level, as is normal. For such patients, supplemental oxygen therapy should be provided cautiously because it may depress the stimulus to breathe, further increasing $PaCO_2$.

Ask the patient with a cough these questions:
- If the cough is a chronic problem, has it changed recently? If so, how?
- What makes the cough better?
- What makes it worse?
- Is the cough productive?

If the patient produces sputum, ask him to estimate the amount produced in teaspoons or some other common measurement. Also ask him these questions:
- At what time of day do you cough most often?
- What is the color and consistency of the sputum?
- If sputum is a chronic problem, has it changed recently? If so, how?
- Do you cough up blood? If so, how much and how often?

If a patient wheezes, ask these questions:
- When does wheezing occur?
- What makes you wheeze?

Grading dyspnea

To assess dyspnea as objectively as possible, ask your patient to briefly describe how various activities affect his breathing. Then document his response using this grading system.

Grade 0: Not troubled by breathlessness except with strenuous exercise

Grade 1: Troubled by shortness of breath when hurrying on a level path or walking up a slight hill

Grade 2: Walks more slowly than people of the same age on a level path because of breathlessness or has to stop to breathe when walking on a level path at his own pace

Grade 3: Stops to breathe after walking about 100 yards (91 m) on a level path

Grade 4: Too breathless to leave the house or breathless when dressing or undressing

- Do you wheeze loudly enough for others to hear it?
- What helps stop your wheezing?
  If the patient has chest pain, ask him these questions:
- Where is the pain?
- What does it feel like?
- Is it sharp, stabbing, burning, or aching?
- Does it move to another area?
- How long does it last?
- What causes it to occur?
- What makes it better?

Chest pain that's caused by a respiratory problem is usually from pleural inflammation, inflammation of the costochondral junctions, sore chest muscles (from coughing), or indigestion. Less common causes of pain include rib or vertebral fractures caused by coughing or by osteoporosis.

Remember to look at the patient's medical and family history, being particularly watchful for a smoking habit, allergies, previous operations, and respiratory diseases, such as pneumonia and tuberculosis.

Also, ask about environmental exposure to irritants such as asbestos. People who work in mining, construction, or chemical manufacturing are commonly exposed to environmental irritants. (See *Listen and learn,* then *teach.*)

KNOW-HOW

Listen and learn, *then* teach

Listening to what your patient says about his respiratory problems will help you know when he needs patient education. The following typical responses indicate that the patient needs to know more about self-care techniques.

"Whenever I feel breathless, I just take a shot of my inhaler."
   This patient needs to know more about proper use of an inhaler and when to call the doctor.

"If I feel all congested, I just smoke a cigarette, and then I can cough up that phlegm!"
   This patient needs to know about the dangers of cigarette smoking.

"None of the other guys wear a mask when we're working."
   This patient needs to know the importance of wearing an appropriate safety mask when working around heavy dust and particles in the air, such as sawdust or powders.

Performing the physical examination

Any patient can develop a respiratory disorder. By using systematic assessment, you can detect subtle or obvious respiratory changes. The depth of your assessment depends on several factors, including the patient's primary health problem and his risk of developing respiratory complications.

A physical examination of the respiratory system follows four steps:
- inspection
- palpation
- percussion
- auscultation.

Before you begin, make sure the room is well lit and warm.

Make a few observations about the patient as soon as you enter the room. Note how the patient is seated, which is likely to be the position most comfortable for him. Take note of his level of awareness and general appearance. Does he appear relaxed? Anxious? Uncomfortable? Is he having trouble breathing? Be sure to include these observations in your final assessment.

Identifying chest deformities

As you inspect the patient's chest, note deviations in size and shape. The illustrations below show a normal adult chest and four common chest deformities.

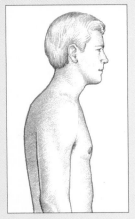

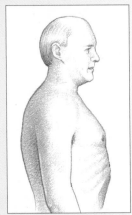

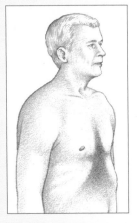

Normal adult chest

Barrel chest
Increased anteroposterior diameter

Pigeon chest
Anteriorly displaced sternum

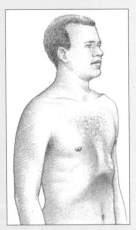

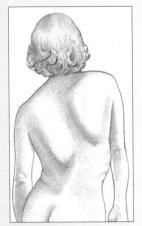

Funnel chest
Depressed lower sternum

Thoracic kyphoscoliosis
Raised shoulder and scapula, thoracic convexity, and flared interspaces

Inspecting the chest

Before you further assess the patient, be sure to introduce yourself and explain why you're there. Then help the patient into an upright position. The patient should be undressed from the waist up or clothed in an examination gown that allows you access to his chest.

Examine the back of the chest first, using inspection, palpation, percussion, and auscultation. Always compare one side with the other. Then examine the front of the chest using the same sequence. The patient can lie back when you examine the front of the chest if that's more comfortable for him.

Note masses or scars that indicate trauma or surgery. Look for chest wall symmetry. Both sides of the chest should be equal at rest and expand equally as the patient inhales. The diameter of the chest, from front to back, should be about half the width of the chest. (See *Identifying chest deformities.*)

Also, look at the angle between the ribs and the sternum at the point immediately above the xiphoid process. This angle—the costal angle— should be less than 90 degrees in an adult. The angle will be larger if the chest wall is chronically expanded because of an enlargement of the intercostal muscles, as can happen with chronic obstructive pulmonary disease.

To find the patient's respiratory rate, count for a full minute—longer if you note abnormalities. Don't tell him what you're doing, or he might alter his natural breathing pattern. Adults normally breathe at 12 to 20 breaths/minute. An infant's breathing rate may reach up to 40 breaths/minute. The respiratory pattern should be even, coordinated, and regular, with occasional sighs. (See *Spotting abnormal respiratory patterns,* page 210.)

AGE ALERT In infancy and early childhood, diaphragmatic breathing is predominant and thoracic excursion is minimal. Therefore, observe the respiratory rate by looking at the abdominal excursion— not the chest excursion. You can also place your hand directly on the thorax to determine the respiratory rate.

An infant's or child's breathing rate is very susceptible to illness, exercise, and emotion, so observe the respiratory rate when the child is asleep or quiet. The respiratory rate can range between 30 and 60 breaths/minute in a neonate, 20 and 40 breaths/minute in early childhood, and 15 and 25 breaths/minute in late childhood.

Watch for paradoxical, or uneven, movement of the chest wall. Paradoxical movement may appear as an abnormal collapse of part of the chest wall when the patient inhales or an abnormal expansion when

Spotting abnormal respiratory patterns

Here are typical characteristics of the most common abnormal respiratory patterns.

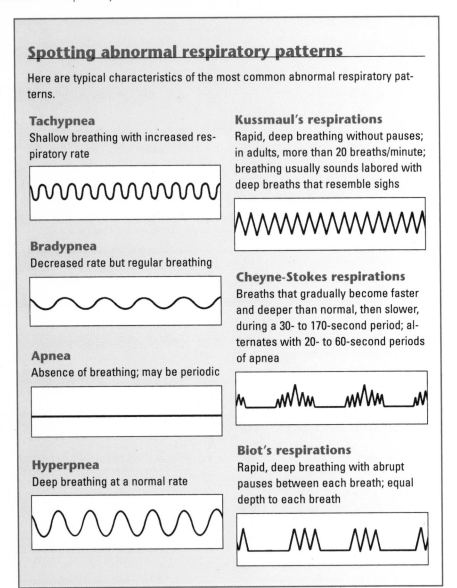

Tachypnea
Shallow breathing with increased respiratory rate

Bradypnea
Decreased rate but regular breathing

Apnea
Absence of breathing; may be periodic

Hyperpnea
Deep breathing at a normal rate

Kussmaul's respirations
Rapid, deep breathing without pauses; in adults, more than 20 breaths/minute; breathing usually sounds labored with deep breaths that resemble sighs

Cheyne-Stokes respirations
Breaths that gradually become faster and deeper than normal, then slower, during a 30- to 170-second period; alternates with 20- to 60-second periods of apnea

Biot's respirations
Rapid, deep breathing with abrupt pauses between each breath; equal depth to each breath

the patient exhales. In either case, this uneven movement indicates a loss of normal chest wall function.

When the patient inhales, his diaphragm should descend and the intercostal muscles should contract. This dual motion causes the abdomen to push out and the lower ribs to expand laterally.

Assessing for clubbing

To assess for chronic tissue hypoxia, check the patient's fingers for clubbing. Normally, the angle between the fingernail and the point where the nail enters the skin is about 160 degrees. Clubbing occurs when that angle increases to 180 degrees or more, as shown here.

NORMAL FINGER

Normal angle
(160 degrees)

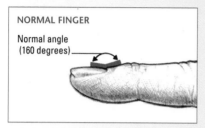

CLUBBED FINGER

Angle greater than
180 degrees

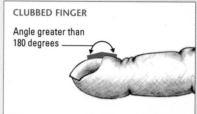

When the patient exhales, his abdomen and ribs return to their resting position. The upper chest shouldn't move much. Accessory muscles may hypertrophy, indicating frequent use. Frequent use of accessory muscles may be normal in some athletes; for other patients, however, it indicates a respiratory problem, particularly when the patient purses his lips and flares his nostrils when breathing.

Inspecting related structures

Inspection of the skin, tongue, mouth, fingers, and nail beds may also provide information about respiratory status.

Skin color varies considerably from person to person, but in all cases, a patient with a bluish tint to his skin and mucous membranes is considered cyanotic. Cyanosis, which results from poor oxygenation to the tissues, is a late sign of hypoxemia.

The most reliable place to check for cyanosis is the tongue and mucous membranes of the mouth. A chilled patient may have cyanotic nail beds, nose, or ears, indicating low blood flow to those areas but not necessarily to major organs.

When you check the fingers, look for clubbing, a possible sign of long-term hypoxia. A fingernail normally enters the skin at an angle of less than 180 degrees. When clubbing occurs, the angle is greater than or equal to 180 degrees (See *Assessing for clubbing.*)

Performing chest palpation

To palpate the chest, place the palm of your hand (or hands) lightly over the thorax, as shown below left. Palpate for tenderness, alignment, bulging, and retractions of the chest and intercostal spaces. Assess the patient for crepitus, especially around drainage sites. Repeat this procedure on the patient's back.

Next, use the pads of your fingers, as shown below right, to palpate the front and back of the thorax. Pass your fingers over the ribs and any scars, lumps, lesions, or ulcerations. Note the skin temperature, turgor, and moisture. Also note tenderness and bony or subcutaneous crepitus. The muscles should feel firm and smooth.

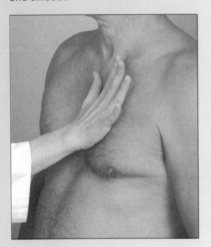 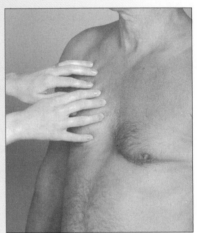

Palpating the chest

Palpation of the chest provides some important information about the respiratory system and the processes involved in breathing. (See *Performing chest palpation.*) Here's what to look for when palpating the chest.

The chest wall should feel smooth, warm, and dry. Crepitus indicates subcutaneous air in the chest, an abnormal condition. Crepitus feels like puffed-rice cereal crackling under the skin and indicates that air is leaking from the airways or lungs.

If a patient has a chest tube, you may find a small amount of subcutaneous air around the insertion site. If the patient has no chest tube or the area of crepitus is getting larger, alert the practitioner immediately.

Checking for tactile fremitus

When you check the back of the thorax for tactile fremitus, ask the patient to fold his arms across his chest. This movement shifts the scapulae out of the way.

What to do
Check for tactile fremitus by lightly placing your open palms on both sides of the patient's back, as shown, without touching his back with your fingers. Ask the patient to repeat the phrase "ninety-nine" loud enough to produce palpable vibrations. Then palpate the front of the chest using the same hand positions.

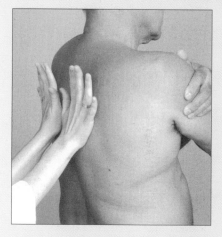

What the results mean
Vibrations that feel more intense on one side than the other indicate tissue consolidation on that side. Less-intense vibrations may indicate emphysema, pneumothorax, or pleural effusion. Faint or no vibrations in the upper posterior thorax may indicate bronchial obstruction or a fluid-filled pleural space.

Gentle palpation shouldn't cause the patient pain. If the patient complains of chest pain, try to find a painful area on the chest wall. Painful costochondral joints are typically located at the midclavicular line or next to the sternum. Rib or vertebral fractures are quite painful over the fracture, although pain may radiate around the chest as well. Pain may also be caused by sore muscles as a result of protracted coughing. A collapsed lung may also cause pain.

Palpate for tactile fremitus, palpable vibrations caused by the transmission of air through the bronchopulmonary system. Fremitus is decreased over areas where pleural fluid collects, at times when the patient speaks softly, and within pneumothorax, atelectasis, and emphysema. Fremitus is increased normally over the large bronchial tubes and abnormally over areas in which alveoli are filled with fluid or exudate, as happens in pneumonia. (See *Checking for tactile fremitus*.)

To evaluate the patient's chest wall symmetry and expansion, place your hands on the front of the chest wall with your thumbs touching

Performing chest percussion

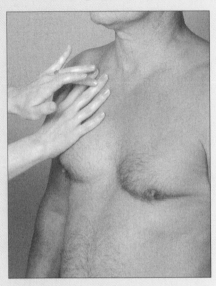

To percuss the chest, hyperextend the middle finger of your left hand if you're right-handed or the middle finger of your right hand if you're left-handed. Place your hand firmly on the patient's chest. Use the tip of the middle finger of your dominant hand to tap on the middle finger of your other hand just below the distal joint, as shown.

The movement should come from the wrist of your dominant hand, not your elbow or upper arm. Keep the fingernail you use for tapping trimmed. Follow the standard percussion sequence over the front and back chest walls.

each other at the second intercostal space. As the patient inhales deeply, watch your thumbs. They should separate simultaneously and equally to a distance several centimeters away from the sternum.

Repeat the measurement at the fifth intercostal space. The same measurement may be made on the back of the chest near the 10th rib.

The patient's chest may expand asymmetrically if he has pleural effusion, atelectasis, pneumonia, or pneumothorax. Chest expansion may be decreased at the level of the diaphragm if the patient has emphysema, respiratory depression, diaphragm paralysis, atelectasis, obesity, or ascites.

Percussing the chest

Percuss the chest to find the boundaries of the lungs, to determine whether the lungs are filled with air or fluid or solid material, and to evaluate the distance the diaphragm travels between the patient's inhalation and exhalation. (See *Performing chest percussion.*)

Percussion sounds

Use this table to get more comfortable with percussion and to help interpret percussion sounds quickly. Learn the different percussion sounds by practicing.

SOUND	DESCRIPTION	CLINICAL SIGNIFICANCE
Flat	Short, soft, high-pitched, extremely dull, found over the thigh	Consolidation, as in atelectasis and extensive pleural effusion
Dull	Medium in intensity and pitch, moderate length, thudlike, found over the liver	Solid area, as in pleural effusion
Resonant	Long, loud, low-pitched, hollow	Normal lung tissue
Hyperresonant	Very loud, lower-pitched, found over the stomach	Hyperinflated lung, as in emphysema or pneumothorax
Tympanic	Loud, high-pitched, moderate length, musical, drumlike, found over a puffed-out cheek	Air collection, as in a gastric air bubble or air in the intestines.

Percussion allows you to assess structures as deep as 3″ (7.6 cm). You'll hear different percussion sounds in different areas of the chest. (See *Percussion sounds.*)

You may also hear different sounds after certain treatments. For example, if your patient has atelectasis and you percuss his chest before chest physiotherapy, you'll hear a high-pitched, dull, soft sound. After physiotherapy, you should hear a low-pitched, hollow sound. In all cases, make sure you use other assessment techniques to confirm percussion findings.

KNOW-HOW **Double-check percussion findings.** *Use other assessment findings to verify the results of respiratory percussion. For example, if an X-ray report on a patient with chronic obstructive pulmonary disease indicates findings consistent with emphysema, you should hear low-pitched, loud booming sounds when you percuss the chest.*

You'll hear resonant sounds over normal lung tissue, which you should find over most of the chest. In the left front chest from the third or fourth intercostal space at the sternum to the third or fourth intercostal space at the midclavicular line, you should hear a dull sound. Percussion is dull there because that's the space occupied by the heart.

Percussion sequences

Follow these percussion sequences to differentiate normal and abnormal sounds in the patient's lungs. Remember to compare sound variations from one side with the other. Carefully describe abnormal sounds you hear, and include their locations. Follow the same sequences for auscultation.

ANTERIOR

POSTERIOR

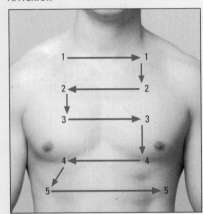
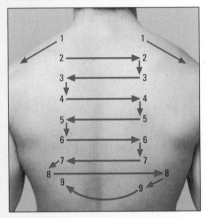

Resonance resumes at the sixth intercostal space. The sequence of sounds in the back is slightly different. (See *Percussion sequences.*)

When you hear hyperresonance during percussion, it means that you've found an area of increased air in the lung or pleural space. Expect hyperresonance with pneumothorax, acute asthma, bullous emphysema (large holes in the lungs from alveolar destruction), or gastric distention that pushes up on the diaphragm.

When you hear abnormal dullness, it means that you've found areas of decreased air in the lungs. Expect abnormal dullness in the presence of pleural fluid, consolidation, atelectasis, or a tumor.

Percussion also allows you to assess how much the diaphragm moves during inspiration and expiration. The normal diaphragm descends 1¼" to 2" (3 to 5 cm) when the patient inhales. The diaphragm doesn't move as far in patients with emphysema, respiratory depression, diaphragm paralysis, atelectasis, obesity, or ascites. (See *Measuring diaphragm movement.*)

Measuring diaphragm movement

You can measure how much the diaphragm moves by asking the patient to exhale. Percuss the back on one side to locate the upper edge of the diaphragm, the point at which normal lung resonance changes to dullness, as shown below left. Use a pen to mark the spot indicating the position of the diaphragm at full expiration on that side of the back.

Then ask the patient to inhale as deeply as possible. Percuss the back when the patient has breathed in fully until you locate the diaphragm. Use the pen to mark this spot as well. Repeat on the opposite side of the back.

Measure

Use a ruler or tape measure to determine the distance between the marks, as shown below right. The distance, normally 1¼" to 2" (3 to 5 cm) long, should be equal on both the right and left sides.

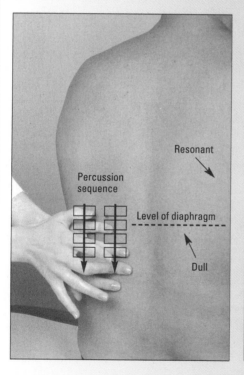

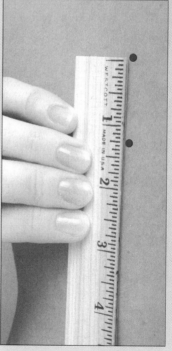

Auscultating the chest

As air moves through the bronchi, it creates sound waves that travel to the chest wall. The sounds produced by breathing change as air moves from larger airways to smaller airways. Sounds also change if they pass through fluid, mucus, or narrowed airways. Auscultation helps you to determine the condition of the alveoli and surrounding pleura.

To gain the most information possible, make sure you perform your assessment in a quiet environment. Also, keep in mind that following a proper sequence and comparing sounds can enhance your assessment findings.

Breath sounds have a wide range of sound frequencies, many near the lower threshold of human hearing. Consequently, the environment for auscultation should be as quiet as possible so that you can hear breath sounds clearly and distinctly. Close the door to the room and eliminate extraneous noises and conversations; turn off televisions and radios. You'll need to develop good concentration skills so that noises from such devices as I.V. pumps, oxygen delivery systems, and ventilators don't interfere with auscultation.

During auscultation, press the diaphragm of the stethoscope firmly against the patient's chest wall over the intercostal spaces. (See *Using a stethoscope.*) Try not to listen directly over bone. Never listen through clothing, which impedes or alters sound transmission. Avoid other extraneous sounds such as those caused by the stethoscope rubbing against bed rails or other objects.

 KNOW-HOW *If the patient has a very hairy chest or back, lightly dampen the chest hair and hold the stethoscope firmly against the skin to minimize the crackling noises produced by dry hair.*

The auscultatory sequence for the posterior chest wall surface includes 10 different sites. (See *Auscultatory sequence,* page 220.) The first site is above the left scapula over the lung apex. From there, the auscultatory sequence follows a pattern that progresses downward from the lung apices to the bases. This pattern covers the entire posterior chest wall surface and includes a comparison of sounds heard over the same auscultatory site over both the right and left lungs. Sites 5, 7, and 10 are located over the lateral chest wall surfaces.

The anterior chest wall auscultatory sequence includes nine sites and follows the same pattern as the posterior chest wall sequence. The pattern also includes sites over the lateral chest wall surfaces.

If the patient is alert and healthy, begin auscultation with the patient sitting upright and leaning slightly forward. Position yourself be-

Using a stethoscope

Proper stethoscope use is important for respiratory assessment. The stethoscope allows you to hear breath sounds transmitted through the chest wall. Most stethoscopes have a diaphragm and a bell, with one or two tubes leading to the binaural headpiece and earpieces. The diaphragm is used to listen for high-pitched breath sounds; the bell is used to listen for low-pitched breath sounds. Applying the stethoscope firmly to the chest wall amplifies high-frequency sounds. However, if too much pressure is applied when using the bell, the stretched skin functions as a diaphragm and filters out low-pitched sounds.

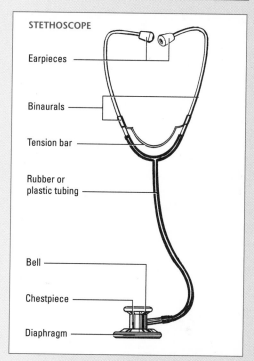

STETHOSCOPE

Earpieces

Binaurals

Tension bar

Rubber or plastic tubing

Bell

Chestpiece

Diaphragm

Checking the equipment

The stethoscope tubing should be no longer than 10″ to 12″ (25 to 30 cm). It should be tightly attached to the binaural headpiece and the stethoscope body to prevent air leakage, which could result in the loss of sound energy. The earpieces must be securely attached to the binaural headpiece, which removes extraneous noise from the environment, to avoid any sound loss. They should fit tightly and should be placed into the ears in an anterior direction so that they conform to the direction of the ear canals. Check the stethoscope to ensure that the diaphragm and bell are locked into place prior to auscultating. Some stethoscopes have a rotating bell or diaphragm that may become disengaged; this can block or muffle breath sounds.

hind the patient. Ask the patient to breathe through an open mouth, slightly deeper than usual, through several respiratory cycles. (*Note:* If the patient is extremely dyspneic, don't ask him to take deeper

Auscultatory sequence

ANTERIOR VIEW

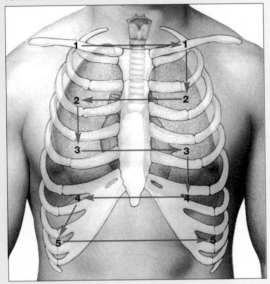

Follow these auscultation sequences to distinguish between normal and abnormal sounds in the patient's lungs. Remember to compare sound variations from one side with the other as you proceed. Carefully describe abnormal sounds you hear, and include locations.

POSTERIOR VIEW

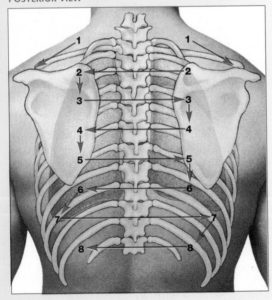

breaths. In this case, begin auscultating for breath sounds at the bilateral lung bases.)

Place the diaphragm of the stethoscope over the left lung apex, and listen for at least one complete respiratory cycle. Then move the diaphragm to the same site over the right lung. Compare the breath sounds heard over these same locations. Continue in this manner, making contralateral comparisons at each auscultatory site.

After you have auscultated the entire posterior chest wall and parts of the lateral chest walls, move to the front of the patient. Have the patient place his arms at his sides and breathe through an open mouth, slightly deeper than usual, as you listen to breath sounds over the anterior chest wall. You can obtain additional information about tracheal sounds by auscultating over the sternum, larynx, and mouth.

KNOW-HOW You may roll comatose, critically ill, or bedridden patients from one side to the other to auscultate dependent lung regions. Listen first over dependent lung regions because gravity-dependent secretions or fluids may produce abnormal sounds that sometimes disappear when the patient is turned, breathes deeply, or coughs.

During auscultation, you'll hear four types of breath sounds over normal lungs. (See *Locations of normal breath sounds,* page 222.) The type of sound you hear depends on where you listen:

■ Tracheal breath sounds, heard over the trachea, are harsh and discontinuous. They occur when a patient inhales or exhales.

■ Bronchial breath sounds, usually heard next to the trachea, are loud, high-pitched, and discontinuous. They're loudest when the patient exhales.

■ Bronchovesicular sounds, heard when the patient inhales or exhales, are medium-pitched and continuous. They're best heard over the upper third of the sternum and between the scapulae.

■ Vesicular sounds, heard over the rest of the lungs, are soft and low-pitched. They're prolonged during inhalation and shortened during exhalation. (See *Characteristics of breath sounds,* page 223.)

If you hear diminished but normal breath sounds in both lungs, the patient may have emphysema, atelectasis, severe bronchospasm, or shallow breathing. If you hear breath sounds in only one lung, the patient may have pleural effusion, pneumothorax, a tumor, or mucus plugs in the airways. In such cases, the practitioner may order pulmonary function tests to further assess the patient's condition. (See *Interpreting pulmonary function test results,* page 224.)

Locations of normal breath sounds

These photographs show the normal locations of different types of breath sounds.

ANTERIOR THORAX

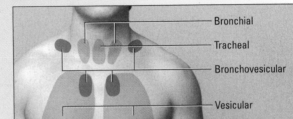

Bronchial

Tracheal

Bronchovesicular

Vesicular

POSTERIOR THORAX

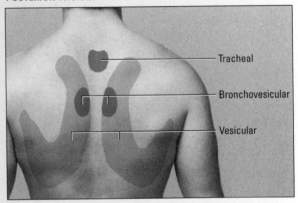

Tracheal

Bronchovesicular

Vesicular

Classify each sound according to its intensity, location, pitch, duration, and characteristic. Note whether the sound occurs when the patient inhales, exhales, or both. If you hear a sound in an area other than where you would expect to hear it, consider the sound abnormal.

For example, bronchial or bronchovesicular breath sounds found in an area where vesicular breath sounds would normally be heard indicates that the alveoli and small bronchioles in that area might be filled with fluid or exudate, as occurs in pneumonia and atelectasis. You

Characteristics of breath sounds

Use this table to help you recognize patterns of breath sounds by their quality, location, and duration of inspiratory and expiratory phases. Note that the thickness of the bars indicates intensity; the steeper an incline, the higher the pitch.

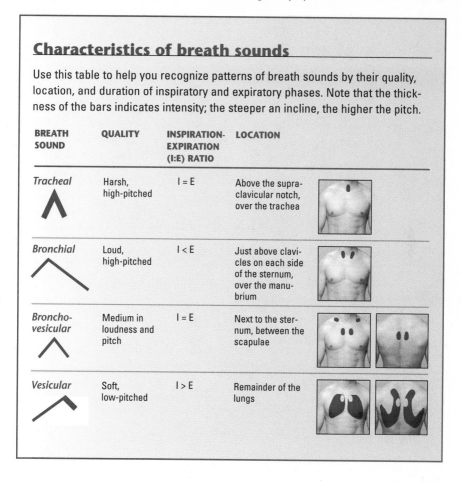

BREATH SOUND	QUALITY	INSPIRATION-EXPIRATION (I:E) RATIO	LOCATION
Tracheal	Harsh, high-pitched	I = E	Above the supra-clavicular notch, over the trachea
Bronchial	Loud, high-pitched	I < E	Just above clavicles on each side of the sternum, over the manubrium
Broncho-vesicular	Medium in loudness and pitch	I = E	Next to the sternum, between the scapulae
Vesicular	Soft, low-pitched	I > E	Remainder of the lungs

won't hear vesicular sounds in those areas because no air is moving through the small airways.

Finally, check for vocal fremitus, which is the sound produced by chest vibrations as the patient speaks. Abnormal transmission of voice sounds—the most common of which are bronchophony, egophony, and whispered pectoriloquy—may occur over consolidated areas. (See *Normal and altered breath and voice sounds,* page 225.)

To check for bronchophony, ask the patient to say "ninety-nine" or "blue moon." Over normal lung tissue, the words sound muffled. Over consolidated areas, the words sound unusually loud. Next, to check for egophony, ask the patient to say "E." Over normal lung tissue, the sound is muffled. Over consolidated lung tissue, it will sound like the letter a. Then ask the patient to whisper "1, 2, 3." Over normal lung

Interpreting pulmonary function test results

You may need to interpret results of pulmonary function tests in your assessment of a patient's respiratory status. Use the table below as a guide to common pulmonary function tests. Keep in mind that a restrictive defect is one in which a person can't inhale a normal amount of air. It may occur with chest wall deformities, neuromuscular diseases, or acute respiratory tract infections. An obstructive defect, in contrast, is one in which something obstructs the flow of air into or out of the lungs. It may occur with a disease such as asthma, chronic bronchitis, emphysema, or cystic fibrosis.

TEST	IMPLICATIONS
Tidal volume (V_T) Amount of air inhaled or exhaled during normal breathing	Decreased V_T may indicate restrictive disease and requires further tests, such as full pulmonary function studies or chest X-rays.
Minute volume (MV) Amount of air breathed per minute	Normal MV can occur in emphysema. Decreased MV may indicate other diseases such as pulmonary edema.
Inspiratory reserve volume (IRV) Amount of air inhaled after normal inspiration	Abnormal IRV alone doesn't indicate respiratory dysfunction. IRV decreases during normal exercise.
Expiratory reserve volume (ERV) Amount of air that can be exhaled after normal expiration	ERV varies, even in healthy people.
Vital capacity (VC) Amount of air that can be exhaled after maximum inspiration	Normal or increased VC with decreased flow rates may indicate reduction in functional pulmonary tissue. Decreased VC with normal or increased flow rates may indicate decreased respiratory effort, decreased thoracic expansion, or limited movement of the diaphragm.
Inspiratory capacity (IC) Amount of air that can be inhaled after normal expiration	Decreased IC indicates restrictive disease.
Forced vital capacity (FVC) Amount of air that can be exhaled after maximum inspiration	Decreased FVC indicates flow resistance in the respiratory system from obstructive disease, such as chronic bronchitis, emphysema, and asthma.
Forced expiratory volume (FEV) Volume of air exhaled in the first (FEV_1), second (FEV_2), or third (FEV_3) FVC maneuver	Decreased FEV_1 and increased FEV_2 and FEV_3 may indicate obstructive disease. Decreased or normal FEV_1 may indicate restrictive disease.

Normal and altered breath and voice sounds

The findings in a normally air-filled lung and an airless lung are summarized below.

	NORMALLY AIR-FILLED LUNG	AIRLESS LUNG, AS IN LOBAR PNEUMONIA
	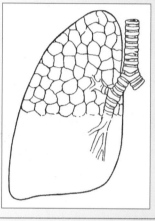	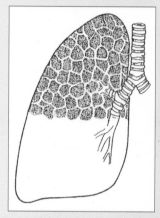
Breath sounds	Predominantly vesicular	Bronchial or bronchovesicular over the involved area
Transmitted voice sounds	Spoken words muffled and indistinct	Spoken words louder, clearer (bronchophony)
	Spoken "ee" heard as "ee"	Spoken "ee" heard as "ay" (egophony)
	Whispered words faint and indistinct, if heard at all	Whispered words louder, clearer (whispered pectoriloquy)
Tactile fremitus	Normal	Increased

tissue, the numbers will be almost indistinguishable. Over consolidated lung tissue, the numbers will be loud and clear.

A patient with abnormal findings during a respiratory assessment may be further evaluated using such diagnostic tests as arterial blood gas analysis and pulmonary function tests.

16 *Breath sound basics*

Breath sounds are produced by air moving through the airways. The diameter of the airway, pressure changes in the airway, and vibrations of solid tissue all affect the sound produced. This chapter discusses the properties that affect airflow and sound transmission as well as the normal and abnormal breath sounds that result. Documenting your findings and structuring an effective care plan are also reviewed.

Understanding airflow

The way air flows through the respiratory system influences the types of sounds heard during auscultation. Understanding airway dynamics and airflow patterns are a key first step in understanding breath sounds.

Airway dynamics

When the chest begins to expand during inspiration, pressure in the pleural space (intrapleural pressure) decreases. The lungs stretch until pressure in the alveoli (intrapulmonary pressure) drops below atmospheric pressure. This change in pressure draws air into the lungs. At the same time, the airways widen, decreasing resistance to the incoming air.

During expiration, the lungs, which were stretched during inspiration, contract. The pressure in the pleural space and the lungs increases until it rises above atmospheric pressure, driving air out of the lungs. As air leaves the lungs, the pressures fall once again. (See *A close look at breathing*.)

A close look at breathing

These illustrations show how mechanical forces, such as movement of the diaphragm and intercostal muscles, produce a breath. A plus sign (+) indicates positive pressure, and a minus sign (–) indicates negative pressure.

At rest

- Inspiratory muscles relax.
- Atmospheric pressure is maintained in the tracheobronchial tree.
- No air movement occurs.

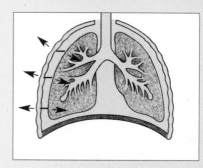

Inhalation

- Inspiratory muscles contract.
- The diaphragm descends.
- Negative alveolar pressure is maintained.
- Air moves into the lungs.

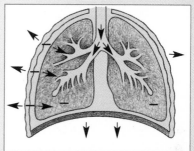

Exhalation

- Inspiratory muscles relax, causing the lungs to recoil to their resting size and position.
- The diaphragm ascends.
- Positive alveolar pressure is maintained.
- Air moves out of the lungs.

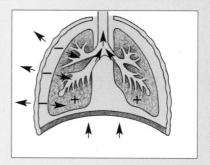

Airflow patterns

The respiratory tract consists of an intricate network of branching airways of various diameters, some of which have irregular wall surfaces. These factors affect the pattern of airflow and the resulting breath

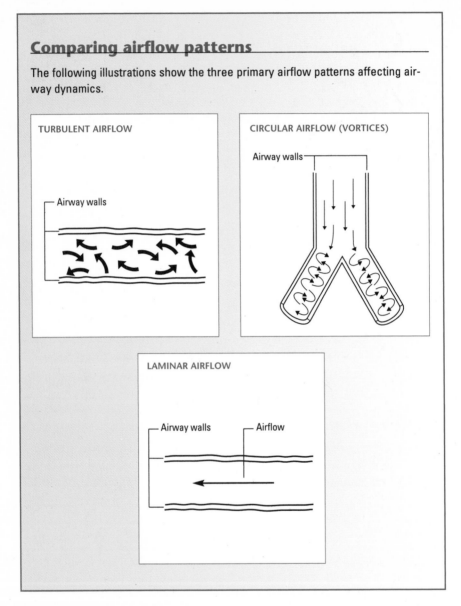

Comparing airflow patterns

The following illustrations show the three primary airflow patterns affecting airway dynamics.

TURBULENT AIRFLOW

— Airway walls

CIRCULAR AIRFLOW (VORTICES)

Airway walls

LAMINAR AIRFLOW

— Airway walls   — Airflow

sounds. Airflow may be turbulent, circular (called vortices), or laminar. (See *Comparing airflow patterns*.)

Turbulent airflow

During rapid airflow movement, air molecules circulate randomly and collide against airway walls and each other, producing an eddying pattern. The colliding air molecules produce rapid pressure changes in the airway, which produces sound. This type of airflow—called turbulent airflow—occurs in the trachea, mainstem bronchi, and other larger airways.

Circular airflow

As air flows into the lungs, it must abruptly change direction in the branching airways. As it does so, it separates into layers, each moving at a different speed. The shearing force of the high-speed airstream against the slower airstream triggers a circular airflow, or vortices. This airflow pattern generates sound as the flow of air carries the vortices downstream.

Laminar airflow

In the small airways and respiratory bronchioles, airflow is slow and linear. This is called laminar airflow. No abrupt changes in pressure or airway wall movements occur to generate sound. Consequently, air movement in these areas produces no sound.

Understanding sound

Mechanical vibrations, sound damping, and impedance matching also affect the sounds heard during auscultation.

Mechanical vibrations

The mechanical vibrations of solid tissue also produce breath sounds. The speed at which these vibrations travel depends on whether they're traveling through air, fluid, or tissue. The frequency, intensity, and duration of these sounds can be measured.

Frequency

Frequency—measured in hertz—refers to the number of vibrations occurring per unit of time. Different frequencies produce the different sounds heard during auscultation. In clinical settings, the term *pitch* is used to describe sound frequency. High-pitched sounds have higher frequencies; low-pitched sounds have lower frequencies.

Intensity

Intensity refers to the loudness or softness of the vibrations that produce breath sounds. Intensity can be measured electronically by recording amplitude. Several factors affect intensity, including the type of structure that's vibrating as well as the distance and type of substance through which the vibrations must travel.

Duration

The duration of the vibrations that produce breath sounds can be measured in milliseconds. However, during auscultation, you'll note sounds as being long or short and as continuous or discontinuous.

Sound damping

Depending on where you listen to breath sounds, certain sounds may be amplified, while others are damped. For example, breath sounds arising from the same location in the lung have a higher pitch when heard at the mouth or over the trachea than when heard over the chest wall. This change in pitch occurs because high-pitched breath sounds are absorbed (damped) as they travel through the lungs and thorax.

Voice sounds are also affected by damping. The resonant qualities of the mouth, nasopharynx, paranasal sinuses, and chest cavity contribute to the pitch and intensity of voice sounds.

Impedance matching

Breath and voice sounds are normally filtered, or damped, when they travel through air, fluid, and tissue. How much the sound is damped depends on how much the substance resists sound transmission. This is known as impedance. When two substances with similar acoustical properties are next to each other, sound is transmitted effectively.

For example, consolidated areas enhance the transmission of breath sounds to the chest wall. This happens because the consolidating substance, such as an inflammatory exudate, collects in alveoli, replacing air with dense tissue. The fluid-filled, airless lung tissue and the chest wall are acoustically well matched, and breath sounds travel more easily. On the other hand, if fluid (or solid tissue) collects between inflated lung segments, an impedance mismatch occurs. Therefore, breath and voice sounds are significantly filtered, reducing the sounds heard on auscultation.

Diseases that increase the impedance mismatch include pleural effusion and empyema. Obesity also causes diminished breath sounds because of the increased distance between the stethoscope and the lungs.

KNOW-HOW *In an obese person, a thickened chest wall increases the distance between the lung tissue and chest wall surface. For better results when auscultating an obese patient's lungs, ask him to take deep breaths through his open mouth while sitting upright or standing.*

Classifying sounds

Both normal and abnormal breath sounds have certain recognizable characteristics. Airflow patterns, regional lung volume, distribution of ventilation, body position, and the site producing the sound all affect the sounds heard during auscultation. In many cases, you can link a normal breath sound to a specific site in the respiratory system. However, this isn't always possible.

Normal breath sounds

Normal breath sounds include tracheal, bronchial, vesicular, and bronchovesicular breath sounds. **(SOUND 51)**

Tracheal and bronchial sounds, which result from turbulent airflow in the first divisions of the large airways, are loud and hollow (tubular) sounding. They're heard best over the trachea and mainstem bronchi throughout inspiration and expiration. **(SOUND 51)** Tracheal breath sounds are described as harsh and high pitched. Bronchial breath sounds are described as loud and high pitched.

Vesicular breath sounds are faint; they're best heard over other chest wall areas throughout inspiration and at the beginning of expiration. **(SOUND 52)** These sounds may result from turbulent airflow in the first few divisions of the large airways. However, because these sounds change with different airflow rates and according to the distribution of ventilation in the lungs, the sounds may also originate in the peripheral airways. It's also possible for vesicular breath sounds to originate in the peripheral airways during inspiration and in the larger airways during expiration. (For more information, see chapter 17, *Normal breath sounds*.)

Bronchovesicular breath sounds are heard over areas between the mainstem bronchi and the smaller airways. They have a pitch and duration midway between tracheal and mainstem bronchial sounds. They're equally audible during inspiration and expiration.

Abnormal breath sounds

Disease processes that alter the airway or airflow dynamics produce abnormal breath sounds. The vibration of solid structures, airflow through narrowed airways, and abrupt changes in airway pressure may all produce abnormal breath sounds. Abnormal breath sounds include adventitious sounds as well as voice sounds.

Adventitious sounds

Adventitious sounds are a specific type of abnormal breath sound. There are two types of adventitious sounds: crackles and wheezes.

Crackles

Coarse crackles (previously known as *rales* or *coarse rales*) are loud, low-pitched, explosive sounds that are discontinuous. **(SOUND 81)** Fine crackles (previously known as *fine rales* or *crepitations*) also sound explosive and are discontinuous, but they have a shorter duration and a higher pitch and are less intense than coarse crackles. **(SOUND 82)**

Wheezes

Wheezes (previously known as *sibilant rales* or *sibilant rhonchi*) are continuous and high-pitched, making a hissing or coughing sound. Wheezes commonly have a musical quality. **(SOUND 83)** Low-pitched wheezes (previously known as *sonorous rales* or *sonorous rhonchi*) are continuous and low-pitched, making a snoring sound. **(SOUND 84)**

You may still see the term *rhonchi* used to describe low-pitched wheezes. The term rhonchi describes a rough, rumbling, low-pitched sound, usually heard during expiration. At times, though, these sounds may be heard during inspiration. Rhonchi, which typically result when fluid or secretions partially block the large airways, may change or disappear when the patient coughs. (See *Comparing adventitious breath sounds.*)

Abnormal voice sounds

Voice sounds are vibrations produced by speech that are transmitted to the chest wall through the tracheobronchial tree. Abnormal transmission of voice sounds may occur over consolidated areas of lung tissue. Voice sounds are classified as bronchophony, egophony, and whispered pectoriloquy.

Voice sounds that have an increased tone or clarity in vocal resonance when auscultated over the chest wall are called *bronchophony*. In a healthy individual, bronchophony is similar to voice sounds heard through the neck. **(SOUND 54)** Voice sounds that are spoken in a normal tone but are transmitted through the chest wall at a selectively amplified higher frequency are called *egophony*. **(SOUND 55)** High-pitched whispered sounds transmitted through airless, consolidated lung tissue are called *whispered pectoriloquy*. **(SOUND 56)** (For more information, see chapter 19, *Abnormal voice sounds*.)

Comparing adventitious breath sounds

The characteristics of discontinuous and continuous adventitious breath sounds are compared in the chart below. Note the timing of each sound during inspiration and expiration on the corresponding graphs.

SOUND	CHARACTERISTICS

Discontinuous sounds

Fine crackles

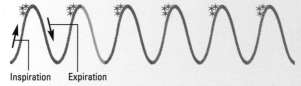

Inspiration   Expiration

- Intermittent
- Nonmusical
- Soft
- High-pitched
- Short, cracking, popping sounds
- Heard during inspiration (5 to 10 msec)

Coarse crackles

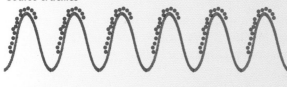

- Intermittent
- Nonmusical
- Loud
- Low-pitched
- Bubbling, gurgling sounds
- Heard during early inspiration and possibly during expiration (20 to 30 msec)

Continuous sounds

Wheezes

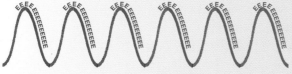

- Musical
- High-pitched
- Squeaking sounds
- Predominantly heard during expiration but may also occur during inspiration

Rhonchi

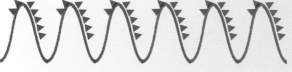

- Musical
- Low-pitched
- Snoring, moaning sounds
- Heard during both inspiration and expiration, but are more prominent during expiration

Documenting auscultation findings

Careful documentation of auscultation findings is essential for determining whether breath sounds have changed over time. After documentation, those findings are used to construct a nursing care plan.

Proper documentation

Be sure to document the location, intensity, duration, and pitch of each auscultated breath in the patient's record. When documenting sound location, use anatomical landmarks, as well as lung bases and apices, as reference points. Note whether you heard the sound over the anterior, posterior, or lateral chest wall surface and whether you heard the sound over one (unilateral) or both (bilateral) lungs.

Describe sound intensity using such terms as "loud," "soft," "absent," "diminished," or "distant." Sound duration refers to the sound's timing within the respiratory cycle—that is, whether it's heard during inspiration, expiration, or both. Timing may be described as early, late, or throughout the respiratory cycle.

Record whether breath sounds have a high or a low pitch. This is especially important when documenting wheezes or crackles. In these instances, a difference in pitch helps differentiate between underlying disease processes.

Here's an example of how to document abnormal respiratory findings: "Late inspiratory fine crackles were heard over the right base posteriorly along the midscapular line, and coarse crackles were heard throughout inspiration and expiration over the left apex anteriorly near the midclavicular line."

Starting a care plan

Your initial assessment of breath sounds provides a baseline for ongoing respiratory assessment and care. After you document your initial auscultation findings, be ready to analyze the data and begin a care plan. As your patient's condition changes, so will the plan. Below you'll find some nursing diagnoses commonly used in patients with respiratory problems. For each diagnosis, you'll also find interventions and rationales. Remember to individualize each patient's care plan using an interdisciplinary approach.

Ineffective breathing pattern related to decreased energy or increased fatigue

This diagnosis commonly applies to patients with such conditions as chronic obstructive pulmonary disease (COPD) and pulmonary embolus.

Expected outcomes
- Patient reports feeling comfortable when breathing.
- Patient achieves maximum lung expansion with adequate ventilation.
- Patient's respiratory rate remains within 5 breaths/minute of baseline.

Nursing interventions and rationales
- Auscultate breath sounds at least every 4 hours to detect decreased or adventitious breath sounds.
- Assess the adequacy of ventilation to detect early signs of respiratory compromise.
- Teach breathing techniques to help the patient improve ventilation.
- Teach relaxation techniques to help reduce the patient's anxiety and enhance his feeling of self-control.
- Give bronchodilators to help relieve bronchospasm and wheezing.
- Give oxygen as ordered to help relieve hypoxemia and respiratory distress.

Ineffective airway clearance related to tracheobronchial secretions or obstruction

This diagnosis commonly applies to patients with such conditions as asthma, COPD, interstitial lung disease, cystic fibrosis, and pneumonia.

Expected outcomes
- Patient coughs effectively.
- Patient's airway remains patent.
- Adventitious breath sounds are absent.

Nursing interventions and rationales
- Teach coughing techniques to promote chest expansion and ventilation, to enhance the clearance of secretions from airways, and to involve the patient in his own care.
- Perform postural drainage, percussion, and vibration to facilitate secretion movement.
- Encourage fluids to ensure adequate hydration and liquefy secretions.

- Give expectorants and mucolytics as ordered to enhance airway clearance.
- Provide an artificial airway as needed to maintain airway patency.

Impaired gas exchange related to altered oxygen supply or oxygen-carrying capacity of the blood

This diagnosis commonly applies to patients with acute respiratory failure, COPD, pneumonia, pulmonary embolism, and other respiratory problems.

Expected outcomes

- Patient's respiratory rate remains within 5 breaths/minute of baseline.
- Patient has normal breath sounds.
- Patient's arterial blood gas (ABG) levels return to baseline.

Nursing interventions and rationales

- Give antibiotics, as ordered, and monitor their effectiveness in treating infection and improving alveolar expansion.
- Teach deep breathing and incentive spirometry to enhance lung expansion and ventilation.
- Monitor ABG values and notify the practitioner immediately if the partial pressure of arterial oxygen drops or the partial pressure of carbon dioxide rises. If needed, start mechanical ventilation to improve ventilation.
- Provide continuous positive airway pressure or positive end-expiratory pressure as needed to improve the driving pressure of oxygen across the alveolocapillary membrane, enhance arterial blood oxygenation, and increase lung compliance.

17 Normal breath sounds

Normal breath sounds result from airflow patterns in the respiratory system, pressure changes in the airways, and vibrations of solid tissues. Various factors influence the sounds heard on auscultation. These include the distance between the source of the sound and the chest wall, the path of sound transmission, and the location of the sound.

Breath sounds are identified by their:
- intensity
- pitch
- relative duration of the inspiratory and expiratory phases.

Listening to normal breath sounds

During auscultation, you'll notice a marked difference in normal breath sounds, depending on where you auscultate. For example, large airways such as the trachea have turbulent airflow, producing loud breath sounds. However, as the air travels throughout the airways and past the segmental bronchi, the airflow pattern changes. Further, the chest wall, pleurae, and air-filled tissue filter the sounds, causing them to diminish. That's why normal breath sounds, heard over most of the chest wall, are soft and low-pitched.

Normal breath sounds include tracheal, bronchial, vesicular, and bronchovesicular sounds as well as the sounds heard at the patient's mouth.

Tracheal and bronchial breath sounds

Turbulent airflow patterns produce the breath sounds normally heard over the trachea (tracheal breath sounds **[SOUND 51]**) and mainstem

Locating tracheal and bronchial breath sounds

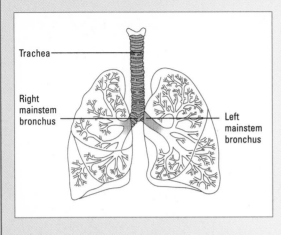

The highlighted portions of this illustration of the lungs show the areas that produce tracheal and bronchial breath sounds.

Trachea

Right mainstem bronchus

Left mainstem bronchus

bronchi (bronchial breath sounds **[SOUND 57]**). (See *Locating tracheal and bronchial breath sounds.*)

Both tracheal and bronchial breath sounds are high-pitched, although the pitch may change, depending on the auscultation site. Tracheal breath sounds are harsh; you'll hear them best over the trachea and larynx. Bronchial breath sounds are loud; you'll hear them next to the trachea and larynx. Use the diaphragm of a stethoscope to auscultate these sounds.

You'll hear these sounds throughout inspiration and expiration, although the sound lasts longer on expiration. **(SOUND 57)** You may also notice that the sound pauses briefly at the end of inspiration. Specifically, the inspiratory-expiratory (I:E) ratio of tracheal and bronchial breath sounds is 1:2 to 1:3, and the sound frequency distribution is 200 to 2,000 hertz. **(SOUND 57)** (See *Auscultation sites for tracheal and bronchial breath sounds.*)

Vesicular breath sounds

Transmitted through lung tissue and the chest wall, vesicular breath sounds result from changes in airflow patterns. You'll hear them throughout the chest (except over the upper sternum and between the

Auscultation sites for tracheal and bronchial breath sounds

To hear tracheal and bronchial breath sounds, auscultate the patient's chest on either side of the sternum from the 2nd to the 4th intercostal space and the patient's back along the vertebral column from the 3rd to the 6th intercostal space, as highlighted in these illustrations.

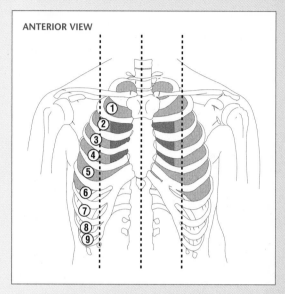

ANTERIOR VIEW

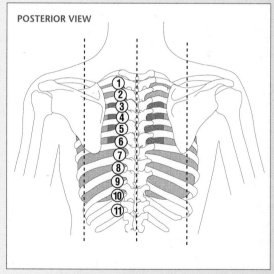

POSTERIOR VIEW

Locating vesicular breath sounds

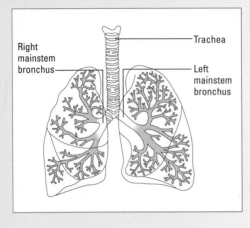

Right mainstem bronchus

Trachea

Left mainstem bronchus

The highlighted portions of this illustration show the airway areas that produce vesicular breath sounds.

scapulae), although they're most audible over the bases of the lungs. (See *Locating vesicular breath sounds.*)

These normal sounds are quieter than tracheal and bronchial sounds, have a low pitch, and make a "swishing" sound. Clearly audible on inspiration, the sounds have a long inspiratory phase but quickly fade on expiration as airflow rates rapidly decline and turbulent airflow moves toward the central airways. The I:E ratio for vesicular breath sounds is 3:1 to 4:1. **(SOUNDS 58 and 59)** (See *Auscultation sites for vesicular breath sounds.*)

Bronchovesicular breath sounds

When auscultating over the large airways, both anteriorly and posteriorly, you'll normally hear bronchovesicular breath sounds. The pitch and duration of these sounds is midway between that of vesicular and bronchial breath sounds. The inspiratory and expiratory phases of bronchovesicular breath sounds are equal, with an I:E ratio of 1:1. (See *Auscultation sites for bronchovesicular breath sounds,* page 242.)

Breath sounds at the mouth

You can also hear normal breath sounds when you listen near the patient's lips. Most likely produced by turbulent airflow below the

Auscultation sites for vesicular breath sounds

The highlighted areas on these illustrations show the best sites for auscultating vesicular breath sounds over the patient's chest and back. Keep in mind that the sounds will be loudest over the lung bases.

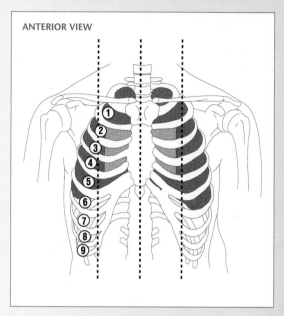

ANTERIOR VIEW

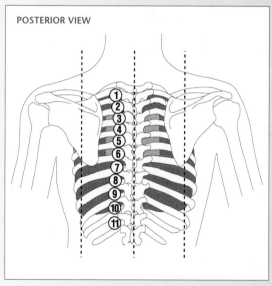

POSTERIOR VIEW

Auscultation sites for bronchovesicular breath sounds

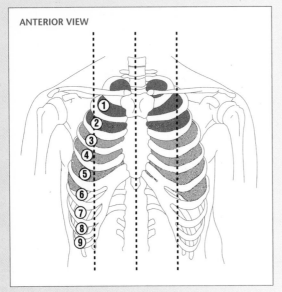

ANTERIOR VIEW

To hear bronchovesicular breath sounds the best, listen to the patient's chest at the 1st and 2nd intercostal spaces or to his back between the scapulae, as highlighted in these illustrations.

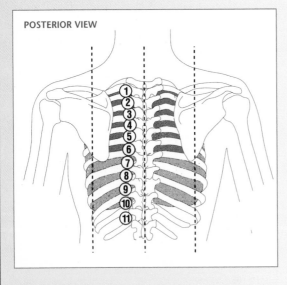

POSTERIOR VIEW

glottis and before the terminal airways, these breath sounds provide a baseline that can be used later to evaluate noisy or paradoxically quiet breath sounds.

The intensity of these breath sounds is as loud and harsh as that of tracheal and bronchial breath sounds. The sounds, which have a moderately high pitch, persist throughout the respiratory cycle.

Evaluating bronchovesicular breath sounds

The intensity of bronchovesicular breath sounds normally changes during deep inspiration and after maximal expiration. These variations typically result from airflow patterns and the distribution of ventilation through the lungs, although variations in intensity may also occur between regions of the lung.

Changes during the respiratory cycle

When auscultating the chest of a patient who's sitting up, you'll notice that bronchovesicular breath sounds are louder over the apices of the lungs during early inspiration and become progressively softer as inspiration continues. **(SOUND 59)** That's because, when the patient inhales while in an upright position, air flows into the lung apices first before flowing into the lung bases, which are in a dependent position.

If you then listen at the patient's back over the lung bases, you'll notice that bronchovesicular breath sounds are initially soft and grow progressively louder with maximal inspiration. You may not notice these changes, however, unless you ask the patient to take deep breaths.

Remember that exaggerated breathing can be tiring for young, elderly, and ill patients. Be alert for lightheadedness or faintness from hyperventilation from deep breathing. Allow the patient to rest as needed.

Changes with the cardiac cycle

Breath sounds heard over the left lower lobe may also vary in intensity during the cardiac cycle.

During systole, when the ventricle contracts, the surrounding lung tissue has room to expand more fully. This increases turbulent airflow to that region and intensifies inspiratory sounds.

On the other hand, during diastole, the expanding ventricle compresses adjacent lung tissue and reduces airflow to that region, which decreases intensity.

Bronchovesicular breath sounds are heard throughout the chest anteriorly, posteriorly, and laterally. Their duration varies, depending on their location, but inspiration is usually followed immediately by a shorter expiration. These sounds have a low pitch that can be heard with either the diaphragm or bell of the stethoscope. **(SOUND 58)**

18 Bronchial breath sounds

Bronchial breath sounds are loud, high-pitched sounds with a hollow or harsh quality. They're normally heard next to the trachea. They're considered abnormal when found anywhere except anteriorly over the large airways.

Bronchial breath sounds occur in abnormal areas when lung tissue between the central airways and the chest wall becomes airless from increased lung density. The dense lung tissue creates an impedance match between itself, the pleurae, and the chest wall. Consequently, sound travels more readily to the chest wall, and the normal filtering of high-frequency sounds fails to occur. The resulting breath sounds are louder and more tubular than normal breath sounds heard over the same area. Also, expiration is significantly louder and longer than normal. The inspiratory-expiratory (I:E) ratio changes from the normal 3:1 or 4:1 to 1:1 or 1:2.

Conditions causing bronchial breath sounds

Conditions that cause bronchial breath sounds include consolidation, atelectasis, and fibrosis, all of which increase lung tissue density because of fluid accumulation, lung collapse, or fibrotic scarring. Bronchial breath sounds occur over the affected lung area.

Consolidation

In consolidation (solidification), fluid, leukocytes, and erythrocytes accumulate in spaces that are normally air-filled, producing a consolidated area. Clinical findings vary, depending on the location of the consolidated area and the causative agent.

The most common cause of lung tissue consolidation is pneumonia, a lung inflammation that can be caused by bacteria, viruses, or chemical insults (as in aspiration).

With classic consolidation, you'll note decreased chest wall movement and dullness to percussion over the affected area. You'll also hear bronchial breath sounds over a dense, airless upper lobe, even without a patent bronchus. **(SOUND 60)** That's because the upper lobe surfaces contact the trachea, and loud tracheal breath sounds travel directly to the dense, airless upper lobe tissues. In contrast, you'll only hear bronchial breath sounds over a dense, airless lower lobe when the bronchi are patent. That's because sound doesn't travel directly to the airless lower lobe tissues.

What you hear

In a patient with lobar pneumonia and right posterior midlung consolidation, you'll hear bronchial breath sounds over the right posterior midlung field. This area is located over the seventh and eighth intercostal spaces along the vertebral column. (See *Bronchial breath sounds in consolidated lung tissue.*)

These sounds are high pitched and have the typical hollow, or tubular, quality of normal central airway breath sounds. They remain audible during both expiration and inspiration, but the expiratory sounds are longer and louder when the patient is sitting up; the I:E ratio is 1:2. These sounds may be auscultated with either the bell or diaphragm of the stethoscope. **(SOUND 60)**

Atelectasis

Atelectasis, which is incomplete expansion of a lung area, is typically diagnosed in postoperative or immobile patients and in some patients with bronchiectasis or pneumonia.

Atelectasis is thought to result from prolonged shallow breathing (hypoventilation) or uncleared secretions that occlude the airway. Because no air enters the distal airways, the segmental or lobar bronchi collapse. If a large airway is occluded, clinical findings include decreased chest wall movement, a dull percussion note, regional changes in lung volume, and bronchial breath sounds over a dense, airless upper airway. **(SOUND 61)** (See *Bronchial breath sounds in atelectasis,* page 248.)

Decreased chest wall movement and lung volume changes may be difficult to detect on examination. If you hear bronchial breath sounds in upper lobes and absent breath sounds in lower lobes, assume a large

Bronchial breath sounds in consolidated lung tissue

The highlighted areas in these illustrations show the location of bronchial breath sounds in a patient with consolidation in the middle of the right lung.

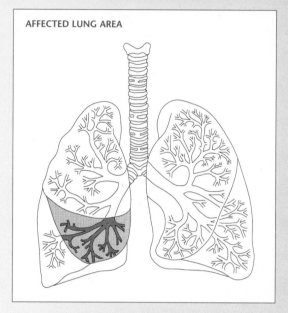

AFFECTED LUNG AREA

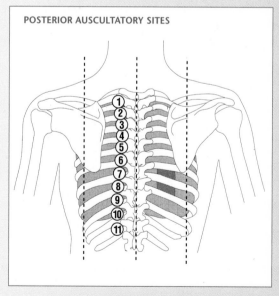

POSTERIOR AUSCULTATORY SITES

Bronchial breath sounds in atelectasis

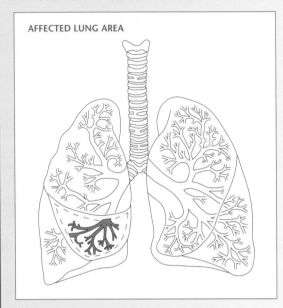

AFFECTED LUNG AREA

Use these illustrations to guide you when auscultating a patient with atelectasis in the right midlung region. The highlighted areas show where you'll most likely hear bronchial breath sounds.

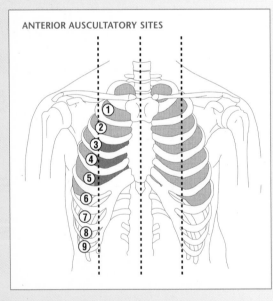

ANTERIOR AUSCULTATORY SITES

airway occlusion is present. Be sure to implement measures to maintain oxygenation and a patent airway.

What you hear

You'll hear bronchial breath sounds over an atelectatic area when the bronchus is patent. You won't hear them over an atelectatic lower lobe if the bronchus is obstructed.

In an unresponsive patient, you'll hear bronchial breath sounds over the right anterior midlung field, located between the third and fifth intercostal spaces from the midsternal line to just right of the midclavicular line. These sounds are high pitched and have the typical hollow, or tubular, quality of normal central airway breath sounds. They're audible throughout inspiration and expiration. When the patient is in the supine position, the inspiratory and expiratory sounds are equal in duration and intensity; the I:E ratio is 1:1. These sounds can be heard equally well with either the bell or diaphragm of the stethoscope. **(SOUND 61)**

Fibrosis

Severe fibrosis (abnormal formation of fibrous connective tissue) may produce bronchial breath sounds that are usually heard over the lower lung regions. Interstitial pulmonary fibrosis is a pathologic change caused by many chronic inflammatory diseases that produce diffuse lung injury.

Some possible causes of pulmonary fibrosis include chronic smoke inhalation and chronic exposure to asbestos. In most cases, however, the cause is unknown. The breath sounds heard over fibrotic areas are similar to those heard over atelectatic areas. **(SOUND 62)**

What you hear

In some patients with asbestosis, bronchial breath sounds are heard anteriorly and posteriorly over both lung bases. Anteriorly, this area extends from the midsternal line to the right and left of the anterior axillary lines over the fifth and sixth intercostal spaces; posteriorly, it extends from the vertebral line to the right and left of the posterior axillary lines over the 7th, 8th, 9th, and 10th intercostal spaces. (See *Bronchial breath sounds in asbestosis,* pages 250 and 251.)

Because the bronchi are patent, bronchial breath sounds heard over fibrotic areas have the typical hollow, or tubular, quality of normal

Bronchial breath sounds in asbestosis

These illustrations highlight the areas where you'll most likely hear bronchial breath sounds in a patient with asbestosis.

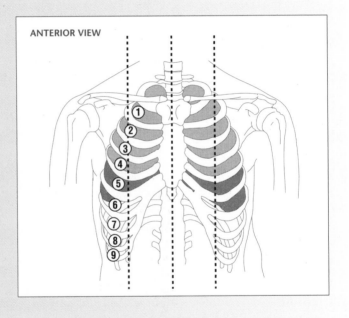

ANTERIOR VIEW

central airway breath sounds. You'll hear them throughout inspiration and expiration.

When the patient is in the upright position, the breath sounds become progressively louder during inspiration and become both louder and longer during expiration; the I:E ratio is 1:1 to 1:2. These bronchial

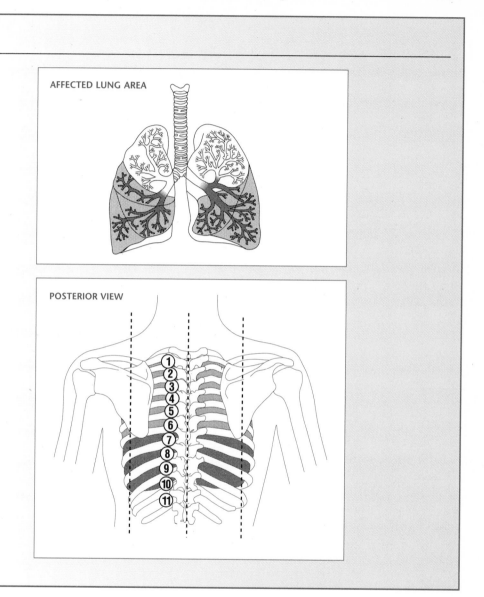

AFFECTED LUNG AREA

POSTERIOR VIEW

breath sounds are high pitched and are heard equally well with either the diaphragm or bell of the stethoscope. **(SOUND 62)**

19 *Abnormal voice sounds*

Voice sounds are vibrations produced by speech that are transmitted to the chest wall through the tracheobronchial tree. Abnormal transmission of voice sounds typically occurs over consolidated areas of lung tissue (areas that have solidified because of inflammation or tumors). Therefore, voice sounds heard during an auscultatory assessment provide valuable clues about the condition of the patient's lungs.

Voice sounds result when air from the lungs passes over the vocal cords, producing vibrations. In turn, the resonance of the mouth, nasopharynx, and paranasal sinuses amplifies these sounds. Healthy, air-filled lungs normally filter high-frequency sounds such as vowel sounds. The pleurae also reflect voice sounds back toward the lung tissue, further diminishing the sounds. Therefore, when you auscultate healthy lungs, transmitted voice sounds should sound like low-pitched, unintelligible mumbles.

On the other hand, consolidated or atelectatic lung tissue enhances sound transmission. When you auscultate lungs with one of these conditions, voice sounds are more distinct. The three types of abnormally transmitted voice sounds are:
- bronchophony
- whispered pectoriloquy
- egophony.

Bronchophony

When you hear voice sounds clearly and distinctly during auscultation, the patient has what's called *bronchophony*. **(SOUND 63)** Occurring over dense, airless lung tissue, bronchophony results from imped-

<u>Consolidation in the left upper lobe</u>

This illustration highlights a consolidated lung area in the left upper lobe. On auscultation, you would typically hear bronchophony in this area.

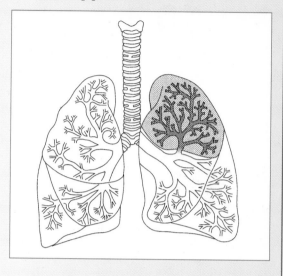

ance matching, which causes high-frequency vowel sounds to travel more easily to the chest wall. Consolidation also increases vocal resonance, which further allows the clear transmission of voice sounds to the chest wall.

For bronchophony to occur, a direct path for sound transmission must exist. For example, you'll hear bronchophony over dense, airless upper lobes because the surface of the lung's upper lobes has direct contact with the trachea. This allows tracheal breath sounds to travel directly to the chest wall. In contrast, for bronchophony to occur over dense, airless lower lobes, the bronchi must be patent, or open. Otherwise, there's no direct path for sound transmission.

What you hear

You'll most commonly hear bronchophony over consolidated areas of lung tissue in the upper lobes. Bronchophony may occur anywhere over the anterior, lateral, or posterior chest wall surfaces. (See *Consolidation in the left upper lobe.* Also see *Auscultating for bronchophony in left upper lobe pneumonia,* page 254.)

To check for bronchophony, ask the patient to say "ninety-nine" several times. Over healthy lung tissue, the words sound unintelligible.

Auscultating for bronchophony in left upper lobe pneumonia

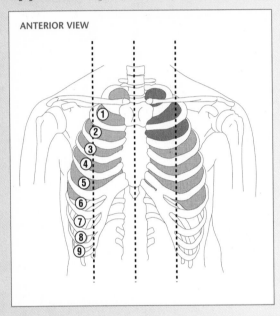

ANTERIOR VIEW

In a patient with left upper lobe pneumonia, which results in consolidation, you'll auscultate intelligible voice sounds over both the anterior and posterior chest wall surfaces. To auscultate the anterior chest wall, listen over the area from just above the clavicle down to the 2nd intercostal space and from the midsternal line to the left of the midclavicular line. To auscultate the posterior area, listen between the 1st and 3rd intercostal spaces from the vertebral line toward the left midscapular line.

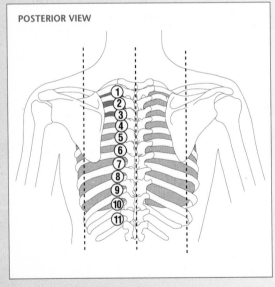

POSTERIOR VIEW

(SOUND 64) Over consolidated areas, the high-frequency sounds are easily understood as words. **(SOUND 65)**

Whispered pectoriloquy

The clear, distinct, whispered voice sound transmitted through airless, consolidated, or atelectatic lung tissue is known as *whispered pectoriloquy.*

In a healthy person, normal lung tissue filters the high-frequency sounds of whispered vowels, making them unintelligible during auscultation. In a patient with consolidation or atelectasis, whispered vowel sounds travel to the chest wall without much filtering, making them audible during auscultation. **(SOUND 66)**

What you hear

You can hear whispered pectoriloquy over areas of dense, airless lung tissue, such as from consolidation or atelectasis. You may hear this voice sound anywhere over the anterior or posterior chest wall surface. (See *Atelectasis in the left lower lobe.*)

Atelectasis in the left lower lobe

This illustration shows an area of atelectasis in the left lower lobe. An area such as this would produce whispered pectoriloquy.

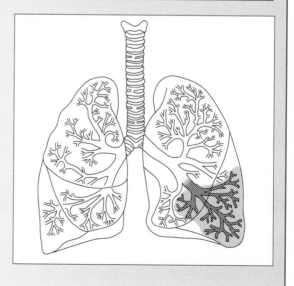

Auscultating for whispered pectoriloquy in left lower lobe atelectasis

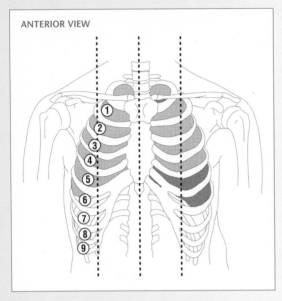

ANTERIOR VIEW

When auscultating the lungs of a patient with left lower lobe atelectasis and a patent bronchus, you'll hear voice sounds over the anterior and posterior chest wall surfaces. To auscultate the anterior area, listen over the 5th and 6th intercostal spaces from the midsternal line to the midaxillary line. To auscultate the posterior area, listen over the 8th, 9th, and 10th intercostal spaces from the vertebral line to the midaxillary line.

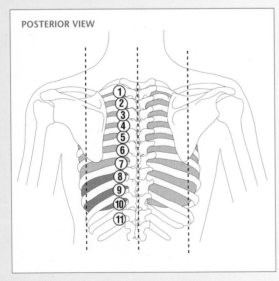

POSTERIOR VIEW

During auscultation, ask the patient to whisper the words "one, two, three" several times. Over healthy lung tissue, the words sound unintelligible. **(SOUND 67)** However, over an area of atelectasis, the high-frequency vowel sounds are easily understood as words. **(SOUND 66)** (See *Auscultating for whispered pectoriloquy in left lower lobe atelectasis.*)

Egophony

Because impedance matching enhances the transmission of breath sounds over areas of consolidation or atelectasis, voice sounds may have a nasal or bleating quality when heard over the chest wall. **(SOUND 68)** This is called *egophony.* Egophony may also occur at the upper edge of a large pleural effusion. (See *Consolidation in the right lower lobe.* Also see *Responding to right lower lobe pneumonia with egophony,* page 258.)

Consolidation in the right lower lobe

This illustration shows a consolidated area in the right lower lobe of the lung. An area such as this would produce egophony.

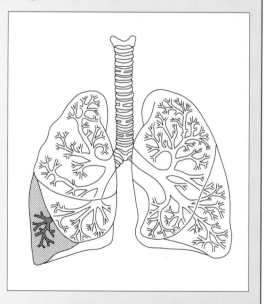

CASE CLIP

Responding to right lower lobe pneumonia with egophony

Mrs. W. was a 91-year-old woman who was admitted 48 hours after an acute ischemic stroke. She had a Dobhoff feeding tube in place. Her file showed that she had dysphagia, altered mental status, and a left-side facial palsy. She had been maintained in semi-Fowler's position. A chest X-ray at admission showed a mild right lower lobe infiltrate and she had required 2 L/minute of supplemental oxygen to maintain an oxygen saturation of 92%. She was started on I.V. vancomycin every 12 hours pending the results of a sputum specimen that was sent for culture and sensitivity.

Over a period of 4 hours, Mrs. W. complained of worsening dyspnea. Her vital signs were:

- temperature: 101.4° F (38.6° C)
- heart rate: 132 beats/minute
- respiratory rate: 32 breaths/minute
- blood pressure: 120/80 mm Hg
- oxygen saturation on 2 L/minute: FIO_2 82%

On physical examination, slight diaphoresis and distress were noted. Cardiac ausculation revealed tachycardia, no murmur, gallop, or rub. Pulmonary auscultation revealed diminished breath sounds at bases, short inspiratory and prolonged expiratory phases, the presence of egophony and dullness to percussion over the right lower lung field.

Concerned that Mrs. W. has impending respiratory distress, the rapid response team (RRT) was called. On arrival, the RRT ordered a portable chest X-ray, obtained a sample for arterial blood gas (ABG) analysis, and followed up on the status of the sputum culture and sensitivity sent the night before.

Mrs. W.'s ABG results were 7.42-40-62-30. A chest X-ray revealed complete opacification of the right lower lobe with air bronchograms. These results explained the finding of egophony as evidence of consolidation of the lung parenchyma, which infiltrates the air spaces with pus. The density of consolidation causes air sounds to be transmitted more clearly than air-filled parenchyma.

As intervention, FIO_2 was titrated up to 5 L/minute to achieve an oxygen saturation of 93%. Mrs. W. was given bronchodilator therapy and aggressive pulmonary hygiene techniques, including chest physiotherapy and a flutter valve to promote airway clearance. Antibiotic coverage was broadened to include a macrolide or fluoroqinolone pending final sputum culture sensitivity.

Auscultating for egophony in right lower lobe pneumonia

In a patient with right lower lobe pneumonia, you'll hear egophony when auscultating the lateral chest wall surface. Specifically, listen over the 5th and 6th intercostal spaces between the anterior axillary line and the midaxillary line.

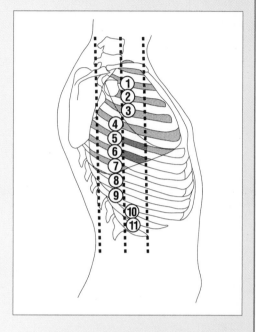

What you hear

You'll hear egophony over a consolidated or atelectatic area on the anterior, posterior, or lateral chest wall surface. (See *Auscultating for egophony in right lower lobe pneumonia.*)

To detect egophony, ask the patient to repeat the letter "E" several times. Over healthy lung tissue, you'll hear a normal sounding "E." **(SOUND 69)** Over consolidated areas, you'll hear a high-pitched sound with a nasal quality, sounding like "A." **(SOUND 68)**

Combined abnormal voice sounds

It's important to know that a constellation of auscultatory findings—bronchial breath sounds, bronchophony, whispered pectoriloquy, and egophony—typically occurs in patients with consolidation. Bronchophony may be easier to hear in patients with pronounced bronchial breath sounds who have consolidation in a single lobe or lung. Whispered pectoriloquy is typically discernible over atelectatic lung segments or areas of patchy consolidation where bronchial sounds or bronchophony isn't completely audible.

20 Absent and diminished breath sounds

Any condition that limits airflow into the lungs causes breath sounds to become diminished or absent. If the flow rate of inspired air slows, less air movement occurs. In turn, airflow becomes less turbulent and the amplitude of breath sounds diminishes.

Diminished or absent breath sounds can also be caused by an impedance mismatch—a condition that occurs when sound travels through two substances that have significantly different acoustic properties. When this occurs, sound transmission is filtered or altered. An example of an impedance mismatch is when sound passes from an air-filled area of lung tissue through a collection of fluid. Sound may also be diminished from increased chest wall thickness, such as occurs in obesity.

Conditions that limit airflow into the lungs include shallow breathing, diaphragmatic paralysis, severe airway obstruction, pneumothorax, hemothorax, pleural effusion, hyperinflated lungs, and obesity. The use of positive end-expiratory pressure (PEEP) during mechanical ventilation may also contribute to diminished breath sounds.

Shallow breathing

When a person breathes normally in an upright position, most of the respiratory movement—and, therefore, most of the ventilation—occurs in dependent regions of the lungs. During shallow breathing, less respiratory movement occurs. Consequently, airflow decreases, resulting in decreased turbulence and, therefore, diminished breath sounds. **(SOUND 70)** (See *A look at decreased turbulence*, page 262.)

A look at decreased turbulence

When breathing becomes shallow, air turbulence decreases. As a result, breath sounds are diminished. These illustrations show the change in turbulence that occurs with shallow breathing.

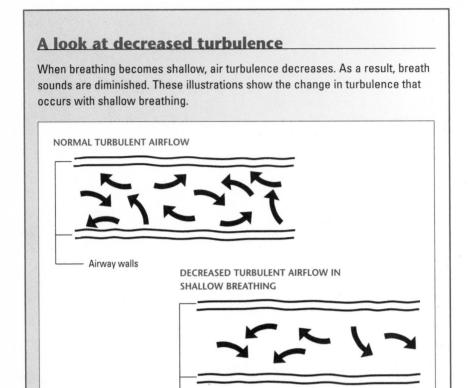

NORMAL TURBULENT AIRFLOW

Airway walls

DECREASED TURBULENT AIRFLOW IN SHALLOW BREATHING

Airway walls

What you hear

You'll hear diminished, softer sounds caused by shallow breathing over the anterior, posterior, and lateral chest wall surfaces. Postoperative patients and patients with rib fractures commonly breathe shallowly because pain limits their depth of respiration. Patients with decreased levels of consciousness from central nervous system injuries or drug overdoses also may have shallow breathing.

Diaphragmatic paralysis

During inspiration, the dome-shaped diaphragm contracts, expanding the lower rib cage, forcing the abdominal contents downward and out, and increasing the length of the lungs. This process lowers intrapulmonary pressure and lets air flow into the airways.

If the diaphragm becomes paralyzed, which may occur after injury to the phrenic nerve, it can no longer participate in normal breathing. The internal and external intercostal muscles, which have a supportive role in normal breathing, must assume control. With only these chest wall muscles initiating the respiratory cycle, ventilation of the lung bases may be limited, resulting in diminished breath sounds.

What you hear

You'll hear diminished sounds caused by diaphragmatic paralysis over the anterior, posterior, and lateral chest wall surfaces. **(SOUND 71)** When caring for a patient with diaphragmatic paralysis and greatly diminished breath sounds, be alert for signs of respiratory distress. Prepare for intubation and mechanical ventilation as necessary.

Airway obstruction

An obstruction in an airway blocks the flow of air and, therefore, changes the breath sounds heard during auscultation. The location of the obstruction determines where you'll hear the changes in breath sounds.

What you hear

If a lobar or segmental bronchus becomes obstructed from, for example, a foreign object or a large mucus plug, airflow stops distal to the obstruction. As a result, breath sounds are absent over the area distal to the obstruction. (See *Lobar bronchus obstruction,* page 264.)

If a mainstem bronchus becomes obstructed, breath sounds are absent throughout the entire affected lung. (See *Mainstem bronchus obstruction,* page 264, and *Responding to mainstem bronchus obstruction,* pages 265 and 266.)

Because the right mainstem bronchus extends from the trachea in a straight line, aspirated foreign bodies are more likely to lodge there. Likewise, endotracheal tubes are frequently misplaced in the right mainstem bronchus. If breath sounds are absent throughout the right lung field after intubation, the endotracheal tube should be repositioned and breath sounds reevaluated.

(Text continues on page 266.)

Lobar bronchus obstruction

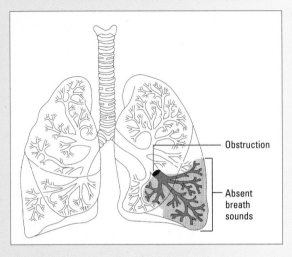

Obstruction

Absent
breath
sounds

Conditions that limit airflow into lung segments—such as a severe airway obstruction—can diminish or even eliminate breath sounds. This illustration shows a lobar bronchus obstruction and the area where breath sounds would be absent.

Mainstem bronchus obstruction

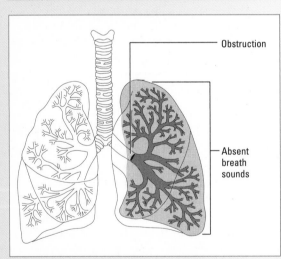

Obstruction

Absent
breath
sounds

An obstruction in the main bronchus stops the flow of air to the entire lung, causing breath sounds to become absent.

Responding to mainstem bronchus obstruction

Mr. H. was a 37-year-old man who had been hospitalized for 5 weeks with multiple traumatic injuries he sustained in a car accident. Having been critically ill, he had prolonged ventilator dependence and myopathy of critical illness. Mr. H. made steady progress and was placed in the rehabilitation unit demonstrating increased activity tolerance and independence with self-care. He had a tracheostomy in place for use with nocturnal ventilation.

Three days earlier, the tracheostomy tube was downsized from a #8 to a #6 fenestrated cannula. A colleague reported that earlier in the day, Mr. H. required endotracheal suctioning for the first time in 10 days. She described the secretions as light green and thick, and she sent the specimen for culture and sensitivity. At the beginning of the next shift, the nurse found Mr. H. to be visiting with his wife and reporting no distress. He was afebrile and his examination was unchanged from the previous day.

Four hours later, Mr. H.'s wife told the staff that something was wrong. On examination, Mr. H. appeared to be agitated and said that he was having trouble getting enough air.

His vital signs were:
- temperature: 99.2° F (37.3 ° C)
- heart rate: 110 beats/minute
- respiratory rate: 30 breaths/minute
- blood pressure: 156/92 mm Hg
- oxygen saturation: 89% on room air.

Cardiac auscultation revealed regular rate and rhythm, tachycardic, no murmur, gallop, or rub. Pulmonary auscultation revealed monophonic expiratory wheezing heard loudest at upper lung fields and diminished breath sounds at bases bilaterally.

Bronchodilator therapy was administered without effect. When it was noted that Mr. H.'s breathing was becoming increasingly labored, the development of stridor was recognized and the rapid response team (RRT) was called.

The RRT drew an arterial blood gas sample for analysis (7.30-46-69-26) and obtained a stat portable chest X-ray that was described as clear throughout with diminished lung volumes, which was no change from the study done 2 days earlier. Mr. H.'s respiratory status continued to decline and the RRT leader called for anesthesia stat.

The anesthesiologist performed oral endotracheal intubation followed by bronchoscopy. Bronchoscopic assessment revealed malacia at the mainstem bronchus distal to the tracheostomy, and a large thick mucous

(continued)

<u>**Responding to mainstem bronchus obstruction**</u> *(continued)*

plug was extracted from the mainstem bronchus at the level of the carina.

Pending the sputum culture sensitivity profile, hydration and empiric antibiotics were started to keep secretions thin and cover nosocomial infection. Mr. H. was managed overnight on continuous positive airway pressure to provide airway stenting and he was referred to an interventional pulmonologist for consideration of endobronchial stent placement via rigid bronchoscopy.

---

*P*neumothorax

Pneumothorax occurs when a tear in the visceral or parietal pleura allows air to accumulate in the normally airless pleural space. (See *Pneumothorax of the left lung.*) An impedance mismatch occurs between the air-filled lung and the collection of air in the pleural space. This causes breath sounds to be significantly diminished or absent over the area of pneumothorax. **(SOUND 72)**

In *uncomplicated pneumothorax*, air enters and leaves the pleural space easily. In certain instances, however, air enters the pleural space with every breath and becomes trapped. This is known as *tension pneumothorax.*

As the trapped air accumulates, it presses on the lung, causing it to collapse. The increasing pressure may shift the mediastinum to the opposite side, causing decreased cardiac output. Unless the intrapleural air is evacuated immediately, this condition may become life threatening, particularly if the patient is being ventilated mechanically.

Signs and symptoms of pneumothorax include sharp, stabbing chest pain; dyspnea; absent breath sounds; inaudible egophony, bronchophony, and whispered pectoriloquy; and increased resonance during percussion. Tension pneumothorax may cause decreased cardiac output, hypotension, and eventually death.

What you hear

Diminished or absent breath sounds resulting from pneumothorax can be heard anywhere over the anterior, posterior, and lateral chest wall surfaces, depending on the location and size of the pneumothorax.

Pneumothorax of the left lung

This illustration (top right) shows pneumothorax in the left lateral lung field, which can be auscultated over the 4th, 5th, 6th, and 7th intercostal spaces between the anterior and posterior axillary folds (highlighted in the illustration below right). When this occurs, you can hear normal breath sounds on the contralateral side over healthy lung tissue. **(SOUND 73)** Breath sounds are absent over the area of pneumothorax.

(SOUND 74) Any diminished breath sounds have a low pitch that's heard best with either the bell or diaphragm of the stethoscope.

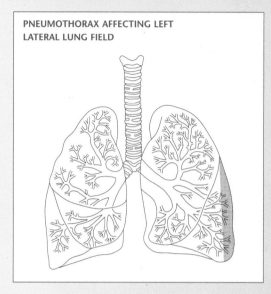

PNEUMOTHORAX AFFECTING LEFT LATERAL LUNG FIELD

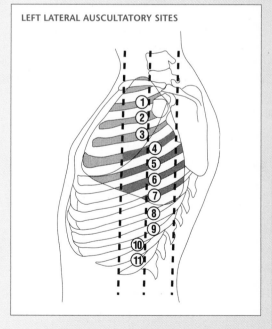

LEFT LATERAL AUSCULTATORY SITES

A small pneumothorax, which may be visible on a chest X-ray, may not alter breath sound intensity enough to be heard during auscultation. A large pneumothorax significantly diminishes or blocks breath sounds.

Pleural effusion

Pleural effusion is the accumulation of fluid in the pleural space. This condition creates an impedance mismatch that causes diminished or absent breath sounds. **(SOUND 75)** (See *Pleural effusion in the right lower lobe.*)

A large pleural effusion compresses adjacent lung tissue, causing atelectasis and producing a dull percussion tone. You may detect egophony, bronchophony, and whispered pectoriloquy at the upper border of the pleural effusion.

What you hear

Diminished or absent breath sounds resulting from pleural effusion may be heard anywhere over the anterior, posterior, or lateral chest wall surfaces, depending on pleural effusion location. If pleural effusion is large, you'll also note diminished or absent sounds over the lower right anterior and lateral chest wall surfaces.

Occasionally, very loud bronchial breath sounds have enough intensity to travel through a small pleural effusion. Be sure to monitor a patient with a pleural effusion for respiratory distress. Prepare for chest tube insertion, if needed.

Hyperinflated lungs

When a lung becomes hyperinflated, it compresses the large central airways. The lung also loses elastic tension, and the airways may have an increased resistance to airflow. These factors limit airflow during expiration, causing decreased breath sounds. (See *A close look at hyperinflated alveoli,* page 270.)

Pleural effusion in the right lower lobe

This illustration (top right) shows pleural effusion in the right lower lung. When this occurs, you can hear diminished breath sounds over the 8th, 9th, and 10th intercostal spaces (highlighted in the illustration below right), from the vertebral line just to the right of the midscapular line. You can hear normal breath sounds on the contralateral side over healthy lung tissue. **(SOUND 76)** The diminished breath sounds have a low pitch that's heard best with either the bell or diaphragm of the stethoscope. **(SOUND 77)**

AFFECTED LUNG AREA

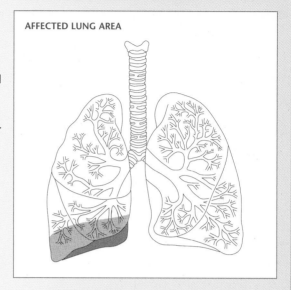

POSTERIOR AUSCULTATORY SITES

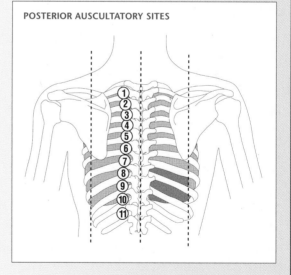

A close look at hyperinflated alveoli

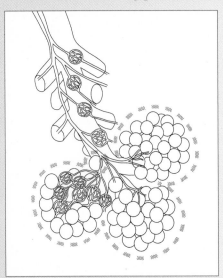

In a hyperinflated lung, air becomes trapped in the alveoli, causing them to become hyperinflated as well.

Effect of PEEP on breath sounds

The use of positive end-expiratory pressure (PEEP) during mechanical ventilation increases functional residual capacity (the amount of air remaining in the airways at the end of normal expiration). Therefore, the lungs remain hyperinflated. Because increased amounts of air in the small airways and alveoli create a mismatch between the pleurae, chest wall, and the hyperinflated lung, breath sounds are diminished. **(SOUND 80)**

Furthermore, the air trapped in a hyperinflated lung creates an impedance mismatch between the hyperinflated lung tissue, the pleurae, and chest wall. This condition further diminishes breath sounds. **(SOUND 78)**

Conditions that cause hyperinflated lungs include chronic obstructive pulmonary disease (COPD), severe asthma, or the use of PEEP during mechanical ventilation. (See *Effect of PEEP on breath sounds.*)

In patients with COPD, the intensity of breath sounds directly relates to the severity of COPD. For example, patients with marked hyperinflation typically have increased anterior-to-posterior thoracic diameters and flattened and immobile diaphragms. The impedance mismatch caused by the trapped air and the decreased flow of air with each respiratory cycle causes diminished breath sounds. Other signs and symptoms of COPD include a hyperresonant percussion note, dyspnea (a primary sign of severe COPD), and inaudible egophony, bronchophony, and whispered pectoriloquy.

When caring for a patient with COPD, monitor his breath sounds. If the sounds progress from diminished to absent, prepare for intubation and mechanical ventilation.

What you hear

In patients with COPD, you'll hear diminished or absent breath sounds throughout inspiration and expiration over the anterior, posterior, and lateral chest wall surfaces. **(SOUND 78)**

If breath sounds are audible, they sound soft with a low pitch. You can hear them best with the diaphragm of the stethoscope. (See *Auscultation sites in COPD,* page 272.)

Obesity

In an obese person, a thickened chest wall increases the distance between lung tissue and the chest wall surface, creating an impedance mismatch. This filters breath sounds as they're transmitted from the pleurae to the chest wall surface. **(SOUND 79)**

What you hear

You'll hear diminished breath sounds over the anterior, posterior, and lateral chest wall surfaces. The location of fat pads determines where the breath sounds are most difficult to hear. For best results when auscultating an obese patient's lungs, ask him to sit up. Then ask him to take deep breaths through an open mouth while you listen.

Auscultation sites in COPD

Because of the wide range of auscultatory findings, you'll need to systematically auscultate the anterior chest wall, lateral chest wall, and posterior chest wall surfaces in patients with chronic obstructive pulmonary disease (COPD). Use these illustrations as guides when auscultating the lungs of a patient with COPD.

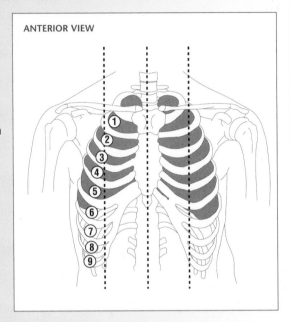

ANTERIOR VIEW

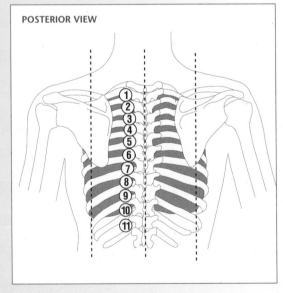

POSTERIOR VIEW

21 *Adventitious sounds: Crackles*

Terms used to describe adventitious breath sounds have changed repeatedly over the years as professionals have tried to describe these sounds more clearly, using more esthetically pleasing words, or by better capturing the acoustic quality or musical tone of these sounds. Currently, adventitious sounds are described according to their acoustic quality, timing, and frequency waveforms. They're further described as being continuous or discontinuous. Continuous sounds include wheezes (previously called *sibilant rales* or *sibilant rhonchi*) and low-pitched wheezes (previously called *sonorous rales* or *sonorous rhonchi*). Remember that the term *rhonchi* is still commonly used in the clinical setting, rather than low-pitched wheezes. These sounds are discussed in detail in the next chapter.

Discontinuous sounds include fine crackles (previously called *fine rales* or *crepitations*) **(SOUND 82)** and coarse crackles (previously called *rales* or *coarse rales*). **(SOUND 81)** Keep in mind that fine crackles vary in intensity, so they may not always sound "fine." To help you better understand these adventitious sounds, this chapter categorizes crackles according to when you'll most likely hear them, such as during late inspiration or during early inspiration and expiration. Pleural crackles, which produce a unique sound, are also discussed.

You'll hear crackles mainly through the chest wall with a stethoscope; however, you may also hear them at the patient's mouth, with or without a stethoscope. Described according to their pitch, timing, and location, crackles are short, explosive, or popping sounds. The characteristics of these sounds change depending on the underlying cause.

KNOW-HOW *When documenting crackles, describe their timing, pitch, intensity, density, and duration:*
■ *Timing means whether the sound occurs early, late, or in the middle of inspiration or expiration.*
■ *Pitch means whether the sound has a high or low frequency.*
■ *Intensity means whether the sound is loud or soft.*
■ *Density means whether the crackles are profuse or scanty.*
■ *Duration means length of time that crackles can be heard during inspiration or expiration.*

Causes of crackles

Crackles may result from air bubbling through secretions in the airways. They also can be caused by a sudden, explosive opening of the airways.

Secretions

In such conditions as pulmonary edema and chronic bronchitis, the trachea and mainstem bronchi fill with sputum. Air bubbling through these secretions causes crackles that you can hear with auscultation. However, because crackles occur mainly during inspiration, and because they may also occur in conditions that produce no sputum, experts think opening airways may cause crackles in the smaller airways.

Airway opening

Normally, peripheral airways in the lung bases close at the end of expiration. These airways stay closed as inspiration begins, allowing air to flow first to the apex of each lung. The small airways distal to the closed peripheral airways remain underexpanded until airway pressures and external forces (such as those exerted with diaphragmatic movement and rib cage expansion) snap the airways open.

The sudden opening of multiple collapsed peripheral airways, along with the resulting explosive changes in air pressures, likely produces crackles. This would help explain why crackles occur over the lung bases of a healthy person who inhales deeply following a maximum exhalation. This is probably also the cause of crackles heard in patients with diseases that cause a restrictive ventilatory defect, such as atelectasis and interstitial lung disease.

Crackles resulting from opening airways have a characteristic loudness and repetitive rhythm, which suggest that the airways open in the same sequence, at the same point in the respiratory cycle, and at the same approximate lung volumes.

You may hear crackles in the lung bases of elderly people and, occasionally, in other healthy people. These crackles clear with coughing and have no clinical significance.

Causes of late inspiratory crackles

Late inspiratory crackles have a high-pitched, explosive sound of variable intensity and density. They're heard most commonly over dependent or poorly ventilated lung regions. Conditions associated with these crackles include:
- atelectasis
- resolving lobar pneumonia
- interstitial fibrosis
- left-sided heart failure.

Atelectasis

Atelectasis is the incomplete expansion of a lung area. It may result from:
- prolonged shallow breathing
- gravitational forces that close airways and deflate the lung bases
- mucus plugging the airways.

It typically occurs in postoperative and immobile patients as well as in those with impaired diaphragm function.

Atelectasis causes poor ventilation in the affected areas and may cause the segmental or lobar bronchi to collapse. If atelectasis occurs in the small peripheral airways, the patient may have no symptoms. If, however, a larger airway is involved, the patient may have decreased chest wall movement, a dull percussion note, and bronchial breath sounds. You'll also hear egophony, bronchophony, and whispered pectoriloquy.

What you hear

Crackles that occur in atelectasis result from the sudden opening of collapsed small airways and adjoining alveoli. These crackles are high-pitched, explosive sounds heard late in inspiration. **(SOUND 85)** Be-

Auscultating for crackles in atelectasis

AFFECTED LUNG AREA

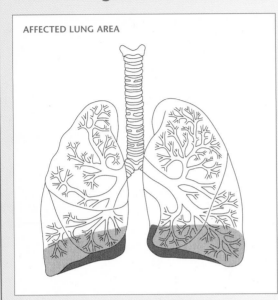

When assessing a post-operative patient who hasn't been coughing and deep-breathing adequately, you may hear inspiratory crackles over the posterior bases of both lungs (shown above left). During your assessment, auscultate between the 8th and 10th intercostal spaces from the left posterior axillary line to the right posterior axillary line (shown below left).

POSTERIOR AUSCULTATORY SITES

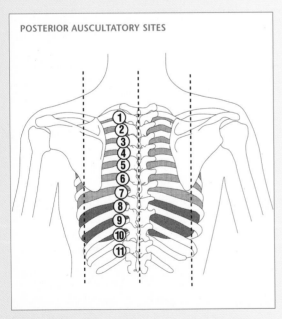

coming more profuse toward the end of inspiration, they vary in intensity.

Because these crackles are poorly transmitted to the chest wall surface, their intensity and density change with only a slight change in stethoscope position. For example, you may hear profuse crackles in the dependent lung regions, but crackles may be scanty or absent in nondependent lung regions. You won't hear atelectasis-related crackles at the patient's mouth. These crackles also clear somewhat with coughing. (See *Auscultating for crackles in atelectasis.*)

The patient's ability to move or ambulate also affects these crackles. Prolonged immobility leads to ventilation of one area of the lung over another, causing atelectasis. (See *Responding to postoperative atelectasis.*)

CASE CLIP

Responding to postoperative atelectasis

Mr. B. was a 40-year-old obese man who had an open cholecystectomy procedure 2 days earlier. During report, his nurse learned that he had a fever of 101.5° F (38.6° C) overnight. Blood and urine samples were sent for culturing, and a chest X-ray was ordered but hadn't yet been performed. Mr. B. had been receiving hydromorphone, pain medication, by patient-controlled epidural analgesia, but the epidural catheter became dislodged the night before and was removed. Since then, the patient had received I.V. hydromorphone as needed.

When the nurse entered Mr. B.'s room, she found him to be anxious, sitting upright, and speaking in short sentences. He said his pain was at "9" on a 0-to-10 scale. He had received 2 mg of hydromorphone I.V. 1 hour earlier.

Physical examination revealed these vital signs:
- temperature: 101.3° F (38.5° C)
- heart rate (HR): 102 beats/minute
- respiratory rate (RR): 26 breaths/minute
- blood pressure (BP): 130/84 mm Hg
- oxygen saturation: 91% on room air.

A cardiac examination showed a regular rate and rhythm, normal S_1 and S_2, a normal sinus rhythm, and sinus tachycardia on telemetry. The patient had diminished breath sounds bilaterally. His surgery incisions were clear and intact. His indwelling urinary catheter was draining to gravity with amber urine output of 50 ml/hour.

Concerned about impending respiratory distress, the nurse called the rapid response team (RRT). The RRT reviewed the situation and ordered

(continued)

Responding to postoperative atelectasis *(continued)*

oxygen via nasal cannula at 2 L/minute, an immediate portable chest X-ray, and insertion of a second I.V. line. The portable chest X-ray showed atelectasis at the bases and no infiltrates. An arterial blood gas analysis performed by the RRT respiratory therapist documented hypoxemia, pH 7.42, $PaCO_2$ – 32 mm Hg, PaO_2 – 79 mm Hg and H_2CO_3 22 mEq/L. Laboratory results were reviewed by the RRT and found to be within normal parameters, with no growth on cultures.

The RRT discussed with the patient and nurse the need for better pain control to improve oxygenation and prevention of pneumonia. Orders included hydromorphone 2 mg I.V. An I.V. patient-controlled analgesia setup was ordered to deliver a basal rate of hydromorphone at 0.5 mg/hour along with a 0.5-mg demand dose with a lockout of 10 minutes. Instructions to the patient regarding use of an incentive spirometer were also given.

Once Mr. B.'s pain was adequately controlled, the nurse urged him to stay out of bed, to use his incentive spirometer, and to ambulate in the hallway. Repeated vital signs revealed:
- temperature: 99.4° F (37.4° C)
- HR: 82 beats/minute
- RR: 18 breaths/minute
- BP: 124/78 mm Hg
- oxygen saturation: 94% on room air.

With better pain control, Mr. B. was able to take deep breaths into the alveoli at the bases of his lungs.

Lobar pneumonia

In resolving lobar pneumonia, many alveoli may still be filled with exudate while surrounding alveoli have higher-than-normal aeration. The air pressure gradient increases greatly in airways leading to the unaerated alveoli.

As these airways snap open in late inspiration, crackles occur. These crackles sound similar to late inspiratory crackles heard over areas with atelectasis; however, these crackles don't change if the patient coughs or changes position. **(SOUND 86)**

What you hear

In a patient with right middle lobe pneumonia, you'll hear late inspiratory crackles over the right anterior chest wall surface between the third and fifth intercostal spaces. (See *Auscultating for crackles in lobar pneumonia.*)

Auscultating for crackles in lobar pneumonia

In a patient with right middle lobe pneumonia, you'll best hear late inspiratory crackles over the right middle lobe (shown above right). Auscultate between the 3rd and 5th intercostal spaces on the right anterior chest (shown below right).

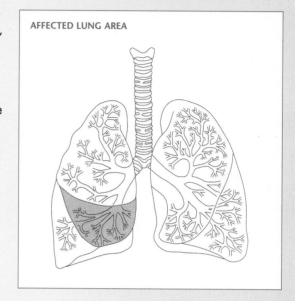

AFFECTED LUNG AREA

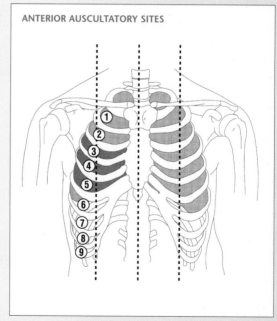

ANTERIOR AUSCULTATORY SITES

Beginning late in inspiration, these crackles are typically high-pitched and become more profuse toward the end of inspiration. **(SOUND 86)**

Interstitial fibrosis

Diffuse interstitial fibrosis impairs or destroys alveoli by filling them with abnormal cells or by scarring the lung tissue. Unaffected alveoli are usually hyperaerated. The lungs become stiff, making inflation difficult, and airflow volumes usually decrease. A patient with a significant amount of lung involvement can have dyspnea and a cough.

During inspiration, the small airways typically open late, causing pressures in the diseased alveoli to fall more than pressures in the healthy alveoli. This increases the pressure gradient, which generates repetitive late inspiratory crackles. **(SOUND 87)** Coughing doesn't affect the profusion of these crackles.

Interstitial fibrosis may be caused by:
- inhalation of heavy metals
- the antibiotic nitrofurantoin (Macrobid)
- some chemotherapeutic drugs
- prolonged inhalation of high concentrations of oxygen.

It also may result from pulmonary sarcoidosis, rheumatoid arthritis, or scleroderma. In most cases, however, the etiology is unknown.

Crackles heard in a patient with known exposure to asbestos may be an early sign of asbestosis, a lung disease characterized by pulmonary inflammation and fibrosis. The longer the exposure to asbestos, the more profuse the crackles.

What you hear

In mild interstitial fibrosis, you'll typically hear crackles at the end of inspiration over dependent lung regions—usually over the lateral lung bases when the patient is sitting up. The crackles may disappear if the patient inhales deeply, holds his breath, or leans forward. However, they usually recur when he returns to an upright position. (See *Auscultating for crackles in interstitial fibrosis.*)

As interstitial fibrosis worsens, you'll hear crackles over both posterior lung bases as well as toward the apices. In later stages of the disease, you may hear crackles throughout inspiration that aren't affected by position changes.

In patients with interstitial fibrosis caused by early asbestosis, you'll hear crackles in the midaxillary area over the lateral lung bases. (See *Auscultating for crackles in early asbestosis,* page 282.)

Auscultating for crackles in interstitial fibrosis

In a patient with mild interstitial fibrosis, you'll usually hear late inspiratory crackles over the lateral lung bases at the end of inspiration. This illustration shows the areas to auscultate.

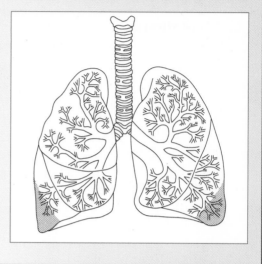

As asbestosis progresses, you may hear crackles over the posterior bases as well as toward the apices. Heard during late inspiration, these crackles have a fine intensity and a short, discontinuous duration. They have a high pitch that's heard best with the diaphragm of the stethoscope.

Left-sided heart failure

Left-sided heart failure leads to fluid accumulation in the lung tissue (pulmonary edema). This narrows the airways, causing them to open late during inspiration. The delayed opening forces pressures to equalize rapidly, resulting in crackles. Common symptoms of left-sided heart failure include rapid, shallow breathing and mild hypoxia.

What you hear

In the early stages of left-sided heart failure and pulmonary edema, you'll hear profuse, high-pitched crackles over the posterior lung bases. **(SOUND 88)** These crackles are inaudible at the mouth.

If pulmonary edema worsens, the airways become flooded with fluid, causing severe hypoxia. At this stage, you may hear low-pitched inspiratory and expiratory crackles at the mouth as well as over the entire chest wall surface. (See *Auscultating for crackles in left-sided heart failure,* page 283.)

(Text continues on page 284.)

Auscultating for crackles in early asbestosis

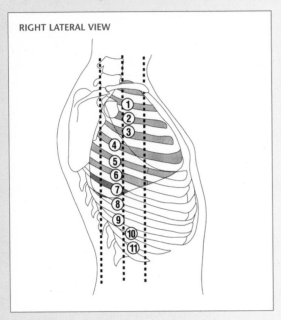

RIGHT LATERAL VIEW

When assessing a patient with early asbestosis, you'll most likely hear late inspiratory crackles over the lateral lung bases. Auscultate over the 7th and 8th intercostal spaces, as shown here.

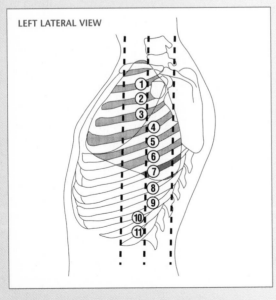

LEFT LATERAL VIEW

Auscultating for crackles in left-sided heart failure

With early left-sided heart failure and pulmonary edema, you'll hear fine, late inspiratory crackles over both posterior lung bases, as shown above right. Focus your auscultation over the 8th, 9th, and 10th intercostal spaces, as shown below right.

AFFECTED LUNG AREA

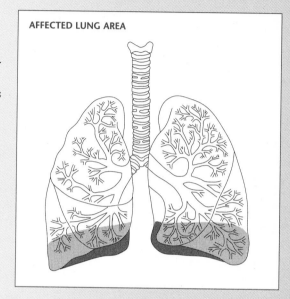

POSTERIOR AUSCULTATORY SITES

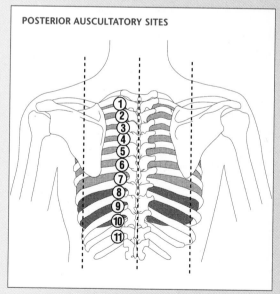

Later, as pulmonary edema worsens, crackles become loud, rattling, and profuse. You'll hear them throughout the chest during late inspiration, with the duration varying according to the degree of left-sided heart failure. The crackles have a low pitch that's heard best with either the bell or diaphragm of the stethoscope, although they may be heard without a stethoscope. **(SOUND 88)**

Causes of coarse crackles

The crackles that occur during early inspiration and during expiration are also called *coarse crackles.* Heard over any chest wall area, these crackles are caused by diffuse airway obstruction. The sound most likely results when the large bronchi intermittently close and when a bolus of air flows past when the bronchi open.

Coarse crackles have a lower pitch than fine crackles. Although they're usually loud, coarse crackles may disappear after the patient coughs, but they're unaffected by the patient's position. Coarse crackles have an irregular rhythm that may be interrupted by short sequences of evenly spaced crackles with the same intensity. Coarse crackles often occur with chronic bronchitis and bronchiectasis.

Chronic bronchitis

Chronic exposure to airway irritants such as air pollution or, more commonly, cigarette smoke, triggers the proliferation and hypertrophy of mucous glands in the airways. This leads to excessive mucus production—as occurs in chronic bronchitis—which causes coarse crackles. Other clinical findings include cough, sputum production, and repeated respiratory infections. Chronic bronchitis can lead to chronic obstructive pulmonary disease. **(SOUND 89)** (See *Lung findings in chronic bronchitis.*)

What you hear

In patients with chronic bronchitis, you'll hear crackles early in inspiration over all chest wall surfaces and at the mouth. (See *Auscultating for crackles in chronic bronchitis,* page 286.) The crackles will be scanty and low-pitched, and they won't be affected by the patient's position. **(SOUND 89)**

Lung findings in chronic bronchitis

This illustration shows the lung areas affected by chronic bronchitis. During auscultation, you'll hear early inspiratory crackles over the entire lung field.

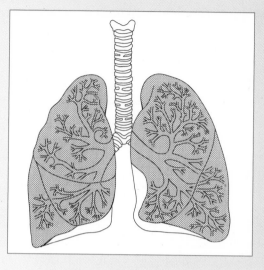

Bronchiectasis

Bronchiectasis is an irreversible dilation of bronchi in selected lung segments. Fibrotic or atelectatic lung tissue surrounds the affected airways, which causes the airways to produce copious amounts of yellow or green sputum. A chest X-ray may reveal old inflammatory changes in the patient's lungs, or more specifically, bronchial dilation and bronchial wall thickening.

Causes of bronchiectasis include:
- foreign body obstruction
- tumor
- viral or bacterial pneumonia (particularly multiple childhood pneumonias)
- chronic inflammatory or fibrotic lung disease
- tuberculosis. **(SOUND 90)**

What you hear

In a patient with bronchiectasis in the left midlung and lower lung, you'll hear crackles over the anterior, posterior, and left lateral chest wall surfaces. (See *Auscultating for crackles in bronchiectasis,* page 287.)

(Text continues on page 288.)

Auscultating for crackles in chronic bronchitis

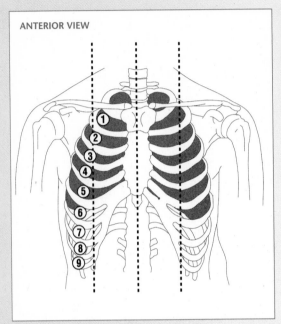

ANTERIOR VIEW

Patients with chronic bronchitis typically have early inspiratory crackles. To hear them, auscultate the areas highlighted in these illustrations.

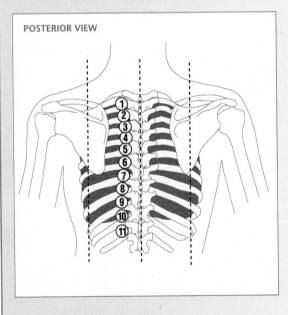

POSTERIOR VIEW

Auscultating for crackles in bronchiectasis

To auscultate crackles in left midlung and lower lung bronchiectasis, listen over the anterior chest wall at the 4th, 5th, and 6th intercostal spaces. Then listen over the posterior chest wall at the 7th, 8th, 9th, and 10th intercostal spaces. These areas are highlighted in the illustrations here.

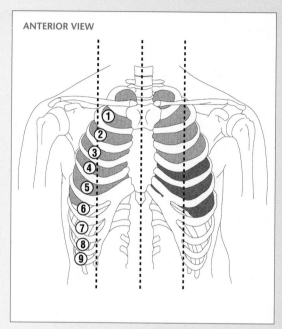

ANTERIOR VIEW

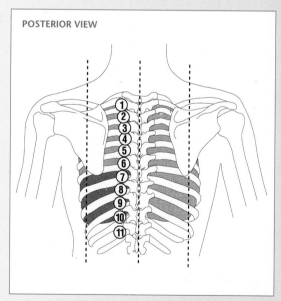

POSTERIOR VIEW

Lung areas affected in bronchiectasis

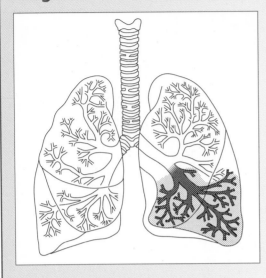

In a patient with bronchiectasis in the middle or lower left lung, you'll hear profuse early to midinspiratory crackles in the areas shown here.

These crackles are profuse, low-pitched, and coarser than those heard with chronic bronchitis. They occur during early inspiration or midinspiration. Although these crackles don't change with the patient's position, the number of crackles you hear may change if the patient coughs. **(SOUND 90)** (See *Lung areas affected in bronchiectasis.*)

Conditions that cause pleural crackles

If the visceral and parietal pleural surfaces become damaged by fibrin deposits or inflammatory or neoplastic cells, they lose their ability to glide silently over each other during breathing. Their movements become jerky and periodically delayed, producing loud, grating crackles known as pleural crackles or pleural friction rub. (See *Auscultating for crackles in pleural friction rub.*) **(SOUND 91)**

You may hear these crackles only during inspiration or during both inspiration and expiration. If fluid accumulates between the pleurae, the pleural crackles disappear.

Patients with pleural friction rub usually complain of sharp pain during inspiration, causing them to splint the affected side to mini-

Auscultating for crackles in pleural friction rub

In a patient with a pleural friction rub in the right midlung, you'll hear pleural crackles over the 5th and 6th intercostal spaces between the right midclavicular and right midaxillary lines. These areas are highlighted in the illustrations here.

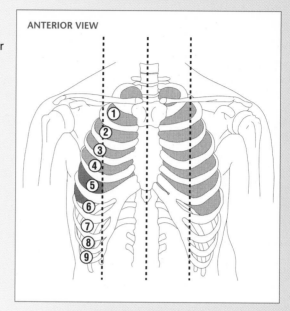

ANTERIOR VIEW

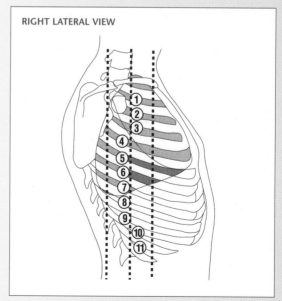

RIGHT LATERAL VIEW

mize muscle movement and chest expansion. Other findings include asymmetrical chest wall movement and rapid, shallow breathing.

What you hear

In patients with pleural friction rub, you'll hear pleural crackles over the affected lung area. Pleural crackles are loud and low-pitched and have a coarse, grating quality. **(SOUND 91)** Their duration is discontinuous.

To distinguish between pleural friction rub and pericardial friction rub, ask the patient to hold his breath; if the rub continues, it's pericardial friction rub.

22 Adventitious sounds: Wheezes

Wheezes are high-pitched, continuous breath sounds with a frequency of 200 Hz or greater and a duration of 250 milliseconds or more. Musical in tone, wheezes result when air passes through an extremely narrowed bronchus. The bronchus walls oscillate between being barely open and completely closed, which produces the audible sound of wheezes. (See *Airflow patterns and oscillations of a narrowed bronchus,* page 292.)

Conditions that cause wheezes include:
- bronchospasm
- airway thickening from mucosal swelling or muscle hypertrophy
- inhalation of a foreign object
- a tumor
- secretions
- dynamic airway compression.

Describing wheezes

When you detect wheezes during auscultation, listen carefully to determine the timing, location, and pitch of these adventitious sounds. These characteristics, which may vary considerably, will reveal information about the patient's underlying condition.

Timing

Describe your patient's wheezes according to their timing in the respiratory cycle. You may hear them during inspiration, expiration, or continuously throughout the respiratory cycle. Also, the patient's wheezes may be episodic (occurring only occasionally), or they may be chronic.

Airflow patterns and oscillations of a narrowed bronchus

Wheezes result when air passes through a narrowed bronchus that oscillates between being barely open and completely closed. These illustrations show the airflow pattern in a narrowed bronchus as well as the airflow pattern in an oscillating bronchus.

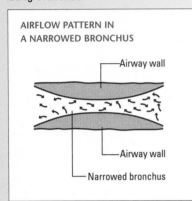

AIRFLOW PATTERN IN
A NARROWED BRONCHUS

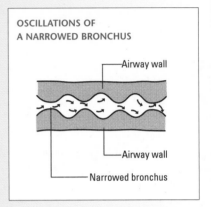

OSCILLATIONS OF
A NARROWED BRONCHUS

Location

Because lung tissue absorbs high-frequency sounds, you'll hear wheezes better when auscultating over the central airways. However, keep in mind that just because you hear a wheeze over the central airways doesn't mean the sound originated there. The airways may simply be transmitting a sound produced in another part of the lung.

Sometimes you'll hear wheezes at the patient's mouth. In fact, if the patient has a severe airway obstruction, you may hear wheezes at his mouth that you won't hear while auscultating his chest wall. If you hear wheezes at the patient's mouth and his breath sounds are reduced or absent, be alert for impending respiratory failure.

Wheezes may be localized to isolated lung areas, or they may be diffuse, occurring throughout the lung field.

Pitch

The pitch, or frequency, of a wheeze can vary widely over a five-octave range. These differences in pitch result from variations in the size and elasticity of the airway as well as the airflow through the narrowed bronchus. Theoretically at least, large, flabby airways generate low-pitched sounds when narrowed; smaller, stiff airways generate high-pitched sounds when narrowed.

Wheezes with different pitches may occur at the same time, or they may overlap. Also, the pitch of a single wheeze may change during inspiration and expiration. During auscultation, you may hear wheezes that produce a single musical note, which may vary in duration and may overlap. These are called *monophonic wheezes*. Other wheezes produce multiple musical tones simultaneously and are called *polyphonic wheezes*.

Understanding types of wheezes

The main categories of wheezes include:
- expiratory polyphonic wheezes
- fixed monophonic wheezes
- sequential inspiratory wheezes
- random monophonic wheezes.

Stridor, which we'll also discuss, is another type of wheeze.

Expiratory polyphonic wheezes

Polyphonic wheezes, which produce several unrelated musical sounds, most likely result from dynamic compression of the large airways during expiration. Because lung compliance and airway resistance don't vary between lung regions, you'll hear these wheezes throughout the lung field. (See *Expiratory polyphonic wheezes*, page 294.)

If you auscultate polyphonic wheezes in a patient who isn't in respiratory distress, suspect a condition causing widespread airflow obstruction, such as chronic asthma or chronic bronchitis. These conditions alter peripheral airway resistance, airway mechanics, and elastic recoil properties throughout both lungs. In turn, this affects the timing of dynamic airway compression of the large airways, which alters the patient's breath sounds.

For example, if a patient with asthma exhales forcefully several times, the central bronchi compress first when elastic recoil of the airways is low or when peripheral airway resistance is high. This compression produces a series of sounds starting with a monophonic wheeze and quickly followed by bitonal sounds. Very soon, you'll hear

Expiratory polyphonic wheezes

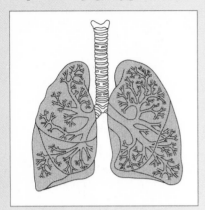

This illustration highlights the lung areas that produce expiratory polyphonic wheezes.

the full complement of sounds that make up polyphonic wheezes through the stethoscope.

Occasionally, you may hear expiratory polyphonic wheezes in a healthy person during forced expiration. In this instance, wheezes result when maximal forced expiration triggers simultaneous dynamic compression of all the airways.

What you hear

To hear expiratory polyphonic wheezes, listen with the diaphragm of the stethoscope over the anterior, posterior, and lateral chest wall surfaces as the patient exhales. (See *Auscultating for expiratory polyphonic wheezes.*)

Loud and widely transmitted, these multiple musical tones begin simultaneously and have a continuous duration. They have a high pitch that remains constant and then rises sharply at the end of expiration. **(SOUND 92)**

Fixed monophonic wheezes

Fixed monophonic wheezes produce a single musical tone of a constant pitch. These wheezes result when air flows rapidly through a large, partially obstructed bronchus. Such an obstruction may result from:

Auscultating for expiratory polyphonic wheezes

When auscultating expiratory polyphonic wheezes, have the patient exhale while you listen over his anterior, posterior, and lateral chest wall surfaces, as shown here.

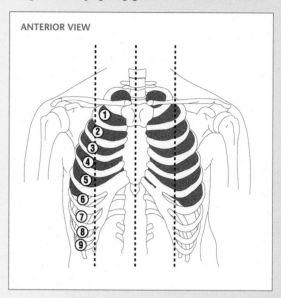

ANTERIOR VIEW

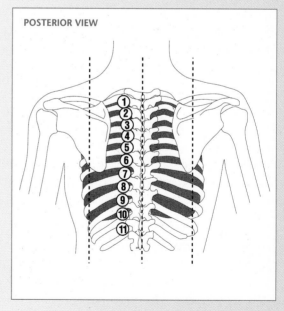

POSTERIOR VIEW

Fixed monophonic wheezes

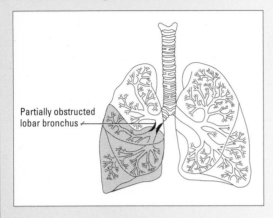

This illustration shows the lung areas that would produce monophonic wheezes in a patient with a partially obstructed lobar bronchus.

Partially obstructed lobar bronchus

- a tumor
- a foreign body
- bronchial stenosis
- an intrabronchial granuloma.

If the patient has bronchial stenosis, the pitch of inspiratory and expiratory monophonic wheezes will vary, depending on the rigidity of the airway. Monophonic wheezes may disappear when the patient lies on his back or turns on to his side. (See *Fixed monophonic wheezes.*)

What you hear

Transmitted throughout the lungs, fixed monophonic wheezes have a low pitch that's heard best with the diaphragm of the stethoscope. **(SOUND 93)** If the patient has a partially obstructed lobar bronchus, you'll hear fixed monophonic wheezes over the anterior, posterior, and lateral chest wall surfaces. (See *Auscultating for fixed monophonic wheezes.*)

Fixed monophonic wheezes are usually loud, and their duration is continuous. You may hear them during inspiration, expiration, or throughout the respiratory cycle.

Sequential inspiratory wheezes

Sequential inspiratory wheezes, which produce a single musical tone, result when airways in unaerated lung regions open late during inspi-

Auscultating for fixed monophonic wheezes

If your patient has a partially obstructed right lobar bronchus, for example, auscultate for fixed monophonic wheezes by focusing over the 3rd, 4th, 5th, and 6th intercostal spaces anteriorly and the 5th, 6th, 7th, 8th, 9th, and 10th intercostal spaces posteriorly. These areas are highlighted in these illustrations.

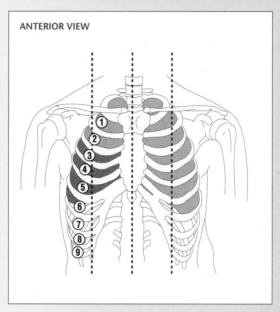

ANTERIOR VIEW

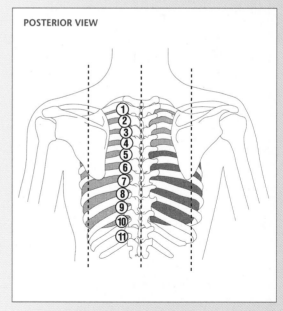

POSTERIOR VIEW

Sequential inspiratory wheezes

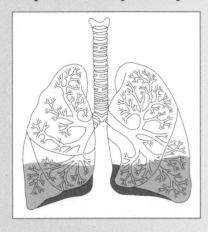

This illustration shows the lung areas where you're most likely to hear sequential inspiratory wheezes.

ration. The rapid inflow of air causes the airway walls to vibrate, generating a series of inspiratory wheezes.

Occasionally, you'll hear sequential inspiratory wheezes over the lung bases of patients with interstitial fibrosis, asbestosis, or fibrosing alveolitis. In patients with interstitial fibrosis, you may hear a single, short inspiratory wheeze—or a brief sequence of monophonic inspiratory wheezes with different pitches—along with the crackles usually associated with this disorder. **(SOUND 94)** (See *Sequential inspiratory wheezes.*)

What you hear

You'll usually hear sequential inspiratory wheezes over the lateral and posterior lung bases. (See *Auscultating for sequential inspiratory wheezes.*)

Sequential inspiratory wheezes have a loud intensity and a high pitch heard best with the diaphragm of the stethoscope. Continuous in duration, you'll hear them throughout inspiration, but they're more predominant in late inspiration. **(SOUND 94)**

Random monophonic wheezes

When bronchospasm or mucosal swelling narrows the airways, single or multiple monophonic wheezes may occur during inspiration, expiration, or throughout the respiratory cycle. Multiple wheezes may oc-

Auscultating for sequential inspiratory wheezes

To hear sequential inspiratory wheezes, auscultate over the posterior chest wall surface at the 8th, 9th, and 10th intercostal spaces (shown at right) and over the lateral chest wall surface at the 7th and 8th intercostal spaces (shown below left and right).

POSTERIOR VIEW

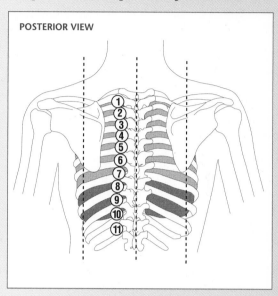

RIGHT LATERAL VIEW

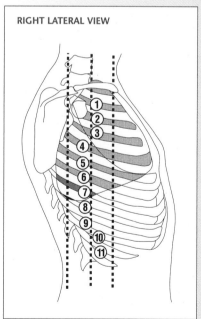

LEFT LATERAL VIEW

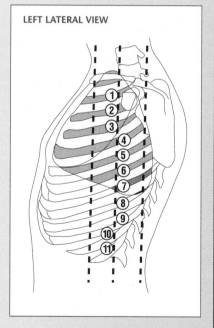

Random monophonic wheezes

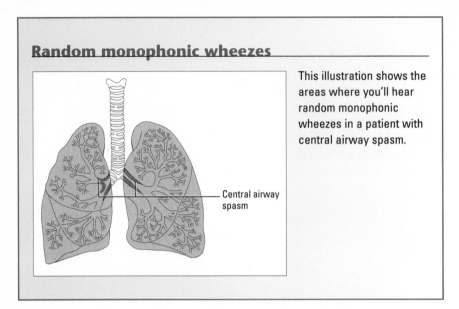

This illustration shows the areas where you'll hear random monophonic wheezes in a patient with central airway spasm.

— Central airway spasm

cur randomly and vary in duration. (See *Random monophonic wheezes.*)

The intensity of the wheeze will vary depending on the area producing the sound. For example, random monophonic wheezes produced in the large central airways are loud and widely transmitted throughout the lung. In fact, you'll hear them at the patient's mouth while standing a distance away. **(SOUND 95)**

In contrast, random monophonic wheezes produced in the peripheral airways are weaker. Because the sounds are filtered as they travel to the chest wall, you'll hear them only when auscultating over the chest wall.

Random monophonic wheezes typically occur in patients with severe status asthmaticus. In status asthmaticus, airway resistance increases. At the same time, dynamic airway compression shifts from the central airways toward the smaller peripheral airways, where the airflow rate is too low to produce airway wall vibrations or sounds.

Status asthmaticus triggers progressive airway obstruction, producing a predictable pattern of wheezing. Initially audible only during expiration, monophonic wheezes eventually occur throughout the respiratory cycle. Because these high-frequency sounds travel through larger airways, you'll also hear them at the patient's mouth.

As status asthmaticus becomes more severe, air trapping and severe airway narrowing force the site of dynamic airway compression to move toward the lung periphery. As a result, all wheezes heard over the chest wall disappear. Called *silent chest,* this phenomenon is commonly accompanied by hypercapnia (an increased blood level of carbon dioxide) and acidosis, both of which are life-threatening.

What you hear

You'll usually hear random monophonic wheezes over the anterior, posterior, and lateral chest wall surfaces. (See *Auscultating for random monophonic wheezes,* page 302.)

Typically loud with a continuous duration, these wheezes have a high pitch heard best with the diaphragm of the stethoscope. They occur throughout the respiratory cycle. Patients with random monophonic wheezes typically have a prolonged expiration.

Stridor

When laryngeal spasm and mucosal swelling contract the vocal cords and narrow the airway, stridor results. (See *Responding to stridor during CT scan,* page 303.)

A very loud musical sound, stridor usually can be heard without a stethoscope at some distance from the patient. The monophonic wheeze of stridor typically occurs during inspiration; however, as airway constriction increases, it may become audible throughout the respiratory cycle. Its intensity distinguishes it from other monophonic wheezes. **(SOUND 96)**

Stridor usually occurs with severe upper respiratory infections. It also may occur with whooping cough, laryngeal tumors, tracheal stenosis, and aspiration of a foreign object.

What you hear

When severe, stridor can be heard without a stethoscope. If the patient has a less pronounced laryngeal spasm, auscultate over the larynx to hear the sound. Very loud with a continuous duration, stridor usually occurs during inspiration but may also occur throughout the respiratory cycle. Its high pitch resembles a crowing sound. **(SOUND 96)**

If the patient with stridor is drooling, the epiglottis may be severely swollen. Because any stimulus may worsen the airway occlusion, avoid examining the patient's mouth. Initiate emergency measures and prepare for intubation. If the edema is severe enough to prohibit intubation, prepare for an emergency tracheotomy.

Auscultating for random monophonic wheezes

ANTERIOR VIEW

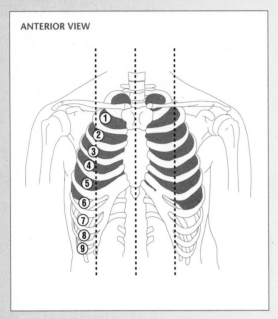

When monitoring a patient for random monophonic wheezes, auscultate the anterior, posterior, and lateral chest wall surfaces, in the areas shown in these illustrations.

POSTERIOR VIEW

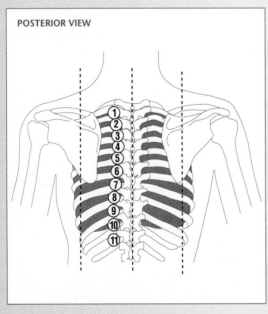

CASE CLIP

Responding to stridor during CT scan

Ms. K. was a 48-year-old woman with chronic obstructive pulmonary disease. She went to an outpatient radiology office for a computed tomography (CT) scan of her chest because a recent chest X-ray revealed a suspicious peri-hilar mass. Ms. K.'s history revealed that she had hypertension and asthma and was allergic to nuts and pollen, but had no known drug allergies. Her daily medications included Lopressor 50 mg every 12 hours and aspirin 325 mg once daily.

Her preprocedure vital signs were:
- temperature: 98.6° F (37° C)
- heart rate (HR): 80 beats/minute
- respiratory rate (RR): 18 breaths/minute
- blood pressure: 152/84 mm Hg.

According to protocol, the nurse placed a peripheral I.V. access hub, gave an ionic dimer contrast dye, and started the scan.

Fifteen minutes later, Ms. K. reported feeling flushed. The nurse interrupted the study and obtained the following vital signs:
- temperature: 98.4° F (36.9° C)
- HR: 110 beats/minute
- RR: 26 breaths/minute
- BP: 110/60 mm Hg.

Ms. K. then appeared restless and was scratching her arms and chest. She said she wasn't nauseated, but she insisted on sitting up so she could catch her breath. As the nurse helped her to a sitting position, Ms. K. developed inspiratory and expiratory stridor. Suspecting an allergic reaction to the contrast agent, the nurse administered 50 mg of I.V. diphenhydramine and called the rapid response team (RRT). When the RRT arrived, they noted that Ms. K. had a reduced level of consciousness. Her vital signs at that time were:
- HR: 160 beats/minute
- BP: 80/50 mm Hg.

They administered epinephrine 0.5 mg I.V. followed by I.V. fluids at 100 ml/hour. Ms. K.'s stridor resolved and she became more alert. She received oxygen via facemask to keep her oxygen saturation above 90% and was transferred to the postprocedure recovery area for monitoring until her vital signs returned to baseline. The nurse explained to Ms. K. that an allergy to contrast dye resulted in a laryngeal spasm and instructed Ms. K. to report this allergy in all future medical interviews.

23 Respiratory disorders

Auscultation skills discussed in the previous chapters are important tools you'll use when caring for patients with respiratory disorders. The disorders introduced earlier are complex; this chapter will help you know what to look for, how each disorder is treated, and what to do for the patient.

Acute respiratory distress syndrome

A form of pulmonary edema that leads to acute respiratory failure, acute respiratory distress syndrome (ARDS) results from increased permeability of the alveolocapillary membrane. Although severe ARDS may be fatal, recovering patients may have little or no permanent lung damage.

Causes

ARDS may result from:
- aspiration of gastric contents
- sepsis (mainly gram-negative)
- trauma (such as lung contusion, head injury, and long-bone fracture with fat emboli)
- oxygen toxicity
- viral, bacterial, or fungal pneumonia
- microemboli (fat or air emboli or disseminated intravascular coagulation)
- drug overdose (such as with barbiturates, glutethimide, or opioids)
- blood transfusion (usually multiple)

- smoke or chemical inhalation (such as nitrous oxide, chlorine, ammonia, and organophosphates)
- hydrocarbon or paraquat ingestion
- pancreatitis, uremia or, in rare cases, miliary tuberculosis
- near drowning.

Pathophysiology

In ARDS, fluid accumulates in the lung interstitium, alveolar spaces, and small airways, causing the lung to stiffen. This impairs ventilation and reduces oxygenation of pulmonary capillary blood. (See *What happens in ARDS,* pages 306 and 307.)

Assessment

Assess your patient for the following signs and symptoms:
- rapid, shallow breathing (usually the first sign)
- dyspnea
- hypoxemia
- intercostal and suprasternal retractions, crackles, and rhonchi
- tachycardia
- restlessness and apprehension
- mental sluggishness
- motor dysfunction.

Diagnostic tests

Arterial blood gas (ABG) values on room air show a partial pressure of arterial oxygen (PaO_2) below 60 mm Hg and partial pressure of arterial carbon dioxide ($PaCO_2$) below 35 mm Hg. As ARDS becomes more severe, ABG values show respiratory acidosis, with $PaCO_2$ values elevated above 45 mm Hg. Metabolic acidosis is also present, with bicarbonate values below 22 mEq/L. The patient's PaO_2 decreases despite oxygen therapy.

Pulmonary artery catheterization helps identify the cause of pulmonary edema by evaluating pulmonary artery wedge pressure. It allows collection of pulmonary artery blood, which shows decreased oxygen saturation, a sign of tissue hypoxia. It measures pulmonary artery pressure, and it measures cardiac output by thermodilution techniques.

Serial chest X-rays initially show bilateral infiltrates. In later stages, X-rays have a ground-glass appearance and, as hypoxemia becomes irreversible, "whiteouts" are seen in both lung fields.

(Text continues on page 308.)

What happens in ARDS

The illustrations below show the development of acute respiratory distress syndrome (ARDS).

1. Injury reduces blood flow to the lungs, allowing platelets to aggregate. Platelets release substances—such as serotonin (S), bradykinin (B), and histamine (H)—that inflame and damage the alveolar membrane and later increase capillary permeability.

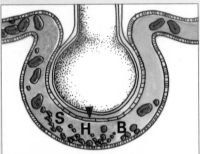

2. Histamines (H) and other inflammatory substances increase capillary permeability, and fluid shifts into the interstitial space.

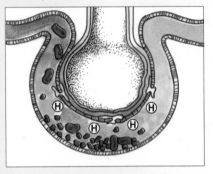

3. As capillary permeability increases, proteins and more fluid leak out, causing pulmonary edema.

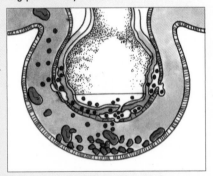

4. Fluid in the alveoli and decreased blood flow damage surfactant in the alveoli and reduce the alveolar cells' ability to produce more surfactant. Without surfactant, alveoli collapse, impairing gas exchange.

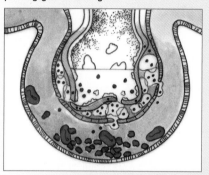

6. Pulmonary edema worsens. Meanwhile, inflammation leads to fibrosis, which further impedes gas exchange. The resulting hypoxemia leads to respiratory acidosis.

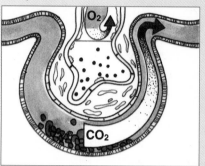

5. The patient breathes faster, but too little oxygen (O_2) crosses the alveolar capillary membrane. Carbon dioxide (CO_2) crosses more easily and is lost with every exhalation. Consequently, both O_2 and CO_2 levels in the blood decrease.

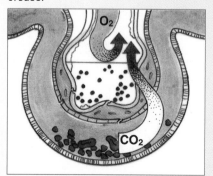

Other tests may be performed to detect infections, drug ingestion, or pancreatitis.

Treatment

Treatment aims to correct the underlying cause of ARDS before it leads to potentially fatal complications.

Supportive medical care includes humidified oxygen through a tight-fitting mask, allowing the use of continuous positive airway pressure. When hypoxemia doesn't respond to these measures, the patient will need ventilatory support with intubation, volume ventilation, and positive end-expiratory pressure. Other supportive measures include fluid restriction, diuretics, and correction of electrolyte and acid-base abnormalities.

Patients who receive mechanical ventilation usually need sedatives and opioids or neuromuscular blocking agents, such as vecuronium or pancuronium, to minimize anxiety. Decreasing anxiety improves ventilation by reducing oxygen consumption and carbon dioxide production.

If given early, a short course of high-dose steroids may be helpful for patients with ARDS caused by fat emboli or chemical injury to the lungs. Treatment with sodium bicarbonate may be needed to reverse severe metabolic acidosis. Fluids and vasopressors maintain the patient's blood pressure. Nonviral infections require antimicrobial drugs.

Patient care

ARDS requires careful monitoring and supportive care. To prepare your patient for transfer to an intensive care unit, follow these steps:
■ Frequently assess the patient's respiratory status. Watch for retractions on inspiration. Note the rate, rhythm, and depth of respirations, and watch for dyspnea and the use of accessory muscles of respiration. On auscultation, listen for adventitious or diminished breath sounds. Check for pink, frothy sputum, which may indicate pulmonary edema.
■ Observe and document the hypoxemic patient's neurologic status. Assess his level of consciousness, and watch for mental sluggishness.
■ Maintain a patent airway by suctioning the patient as needed.
■ Closely monitor heart rate and rhythm and blood pressure.
■ Reposition the patient often, and observe for hypotension, increased secretions, or elevated body temperature—all signs of deterioration.
■ Evaluate the patient. After successful treatment, he should have normal ABG values; a normal respiratory rate, depth, and pattern; and clear breath sounds.

Acute respiratory failure

Acute respiratory failure (ARF) occurs when the lungs no longer meet the body's metabolic needs.

In patients with essentially normal lung tissue, a partial pressure of arterial carbon dioxide ($PaCO_2$) above 50 mm Hg and a partial pressure of arterial oxygen (PaO_2) below 50 mm Hg usually indicate ARF. However, these limits don't apply to patients with chronic obstructive pulmonary disease (COPD), who commonly have a consistently high $PaCO_2$ and low PaO_2. In patients with COPD, only acute deterioration in arterial blood gas (ABG) values, with corresponding clinical deterioration, indicates ARF.

Causes

ARF may develop from any condition that increases the work of breathing and decreases the respiratory drive, including:
- respiratory tract infections (such as bronchitis and pneumonia—the most common causes)
- bronchospasm
- accumulated secretions from cough suppression
- central nervous system depression from head trauma or injudicious use of sedatives, opioids, tranquilizers, or oxygen
- cardiovascular disorders (such as myocardial infarction, heart failure, or pulmonary emboli)
- airway irritants (such as smoke or fumes)
- endocrine and metabolic disorders (such as myxedema or metabolic alkalosis)
- thoracic abnormalities (including chest trauma, pneumothorax, or thoracic or abdominal surgery).

Pathophysiology

ARF results from impaired gas exchange, when the lungs don't oxygenate the blood adequately or fail to prevent carbon dioxide retention.

Any condition associated with hypoventilation (reduced volume of air moving into and out of the lung), ventilation-perfusion mismatch (too little ventilation with normal blood flow or too little blood flow with normal ventilation), or intrapulmonary shunting (right-to-left shunting in which blood passes from the heart's right side to its left without being oxygenated) can cause ARF if left untreated.

Assessment

Patients with ARF experience hypoxemia and acidemia affecting all body organs, especially the central nervous, respiratory, and cardiovascular systems. Although specific symptoms vary with the underlying cause, you should always assess for:

- altered respirations (increased, decreased, or normal rate; shallow, deep, or alternating shallow and deep respirations; possible cyanosis; crackles, rhonchi, wheezes, or diminished breath sounds on chest auscultation)
- cardiac arrhythmias (from myocardial hypoxia)
- tachycardia (occurs early in response to low PaO_2)
- pulmonary hypertension (increased pressures on the right side of the heart, elevated neck veins, enlarged liver, and peripheral edema)
- altered mentation (restlessness, confusion, loss of concentration, irritability, tremulousness, diminished tendon reflexes, or papilledema).

Diagnostic tests

Progressive deterioration in ABG levels and pH, when compared with the patient's baseline values, strongly suggests ARF. (In patients with essentially normal lung tissue, a pH value below 7.35 usually indicates ARF. However, COPD patients display an even greater deviation in pH values, along with deviations in $PaCO_2$ and PaO_2.)

Serum bicarbonate shows increased levels, either because of metabolic alkalosis or from metabolic compensation for chronic respiratory acidosis.

Complete blood count (CBC) reveals low a hemoglobin level and hematocrit (possibly from blood loss), indicating decreased oxygen-carrying capacity. CBC will also show an elevated white blood cell count if ARF results from bacterial infection (pathogens identified using Gram stain and sputum culture).

Serum electrolyte levels reveal hypokalemia, possibly from compensatory hyperventilation (an attempt to correct alkalosis), and hypochloremia, which is common in metabolic alkalosis.

Chest X-rays show pulmonary abnormalities, such as emphysema, atelectasis, lesions, pneumothorax, infiltrates, and effusions.

Electrocardiography discloses arrhythmias, which commonly suggest cor pulmonale and myocardial hypoxia.

Treatment

In COPD patients, ARF is an emergency requiring cautious oxygen therapy (using nasal prongs or a Venturi mask) to raise the patient's PaO_2.

If significant respiratory acidosis persists, mechanical ventilation through an endotracheal (ET) or a tracheostomy tube may be necessary. High-frequency ventilation may be used if the patient doesn't respond to conventional mechanical ventilation. Prone positioning may also prove beneficial. Treatment routinely includes antibiotics for infection, bronchodilators and, possibly, steroids.

Patient care

ARF requires close attention to airway patency and oxygen supply. Follow these steps:

■ To reverse hypoxemia, administer oxygen at appropriate concentrations to maintain PaO_2 at a minimum of 50 mm Hg. Patients with COPD usually need only small amounts of supplemental oxygen. Watch for a positive response, such as improvement in ABG results and the patient's breathing and color.

■ Maintain a patent airway. If the patient is intubated and lethargic, turn him every 1 to 2 hours. Use postural drainage and chest physiotherapy to help clear secretions.

■ In an intubated patient, suction the airways before and after hyperoxygenation, as required. Assess for changes in quantity, consistency, and color of sputum. To prevent aspiration and reduce the risk of ventilator-related pneumonia, always suction the oropharynx and the area above the cuff of the ET tube before deflating the cuff. Provide humidity to liquefy secretions.

■ Observe the patient closely for respiratory arrest. Auscultate for breath sounds. Monitor ABG levels and report changes immediately.

■ Monitor serum electrolyte levels and correct imbalances; monitor fluid balance by recording fluid intake and output and daily weight.

■ Check the cardiac monitor for arrhythmias.

■ If the patient requires mechanical ventilation and is unstable, he'll probably be transferred to an intensive care unit. Arrange for his safe transfer.

■ If the patient isn't on mechanical ventilation and is retaining carbon dioxide, encourage him to cough and breathe deeply with pursed lips. If the patient is alert, teach and encourage him to use an incentive spirometer.

■ Evaluate the patient. Make sure that ABG values are normal, with a PaO_2 greater than 50 mm Hg, and that the patient can make a normal respiratory effort.

Asbestosis

Asbestosis is characterized by diffuse interstitial pulmonary fibrosis. Prolonged exposure to airborne asbestos particles causes pleural plaques and tumors of the pleura and peritoneum. Asbestosis may develop 15 to 20 years after the period of regular exposure to asbestos has ended. (See *A close look at asbestosis.*)

People at high risk for asbestosis include workers in the mining, milling, construction, fireproofing, and textile industries. Asbestos is also used in paints, plastics, and brake and clutch linings. Cigarette smoking increases the risk of asbestosis. In fact, an asbestos worker who smokes is 90 times more likely to develop lung cancer than a smoker who has never worked with asbestos.

Family members of asbestos workers may develop asbestosis from exposure to stray fibers shaken off the workers' clothing. The general public may be exposed to fibrous asbestos dust in deteriorating buildings or in waste piles from asbestos plants.

Causes

Asbestosis results from prolonged inhalation of asbestos fibers.

Pathophysiology

Asbestosis begins when inhaled asbestos fibers travel down the airway and penetrate respiratory bronchioles and alveolar walls.

The fibers become encased in a brown, iron-rich, proteinlike sheath in sputum or lung tissue. Interstitial fibrosis may develop in lower lung zones, affecting lung parenchyma and the pleurae. Raised hyaline plaques may form in the parietal pleura, diaphragm, and pleura adjacent to the pericardium.

Assessment

Asbestosis causes numerous respiratory symptoms, including:
■ dyspnea on exertion
■ possibly dyspnea at rest (with extensive fibrosis)
■ severe, nonproductive cough in nonsmokers
■ productive cough in smokers

A close look at asbestosis

After years of exposure to asbestos, healthy lung tissue progresses to massive pulmonary fibrosis, as shown below right.

HEALTHY LUNG TISSUE

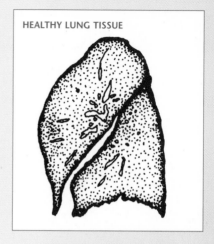

SIMPLE ASBESTOSIS

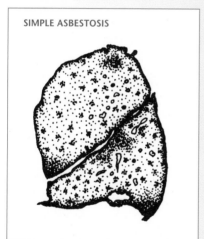

PROGRESSIVE MASSIVE FIBROSIS

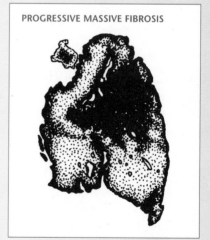

- chest pain (usually pleuritic)
- pleural friction rub and crackles on auscultation
- decreased lung inflation
- decreased forced expiratory volume and vital capacity
- recurrent pleural effusions
- recurrent respiratory tract infections
- finger clubbing.

Asbestosis may progress to pulmonary fibrosis with respiratory failure and cardiovascular complications, including pulmonary hypertension and cor pulmonale.

Diagnostic tests

Chest X-rays may show fine, irregular, linear, diffuse infiltrates. With extensive fibrosis, the lungs have a honeycomb or ground-glass appearance. Other findings include pleural thickening and calcification, bilateral obliteration of costophrenic angles and, in later disease stages, an enlarged heart with a classic "shaggy" border.

Pulmonary function tests (PFTs) may identify decreased vital capacity, forced vital capacity (FVC), and total lung capacity; decreased or normal forced expiratory volume in 1 second (FEV_1); a normal ratio of FEV_1 to FVC; and reduced diffusing capacity for carbon monoxide when fibrosis destroys alveolar walls and thickens the alveolocapillary membrane.

Arterial blood gas analysis may reveal decreased partial pressure of arterial oxygen and partial pressure of arterial carbon dioxide from hyperventilation.

Treatment

Treatment of asbestosis includes chest physiotherapy, aerosol therapy (including mucolytics), oxygen administration, and a high fluid intake of at least 3 qt (3 L) per day. Antibiotics are used to treat respiratory infections. Patients may also require diuretics, digoxin, and salt restriction.

Patient care

Your care will be mainly supportive. Include these measures in your care:
- Initiate measures to relieve symptoms and control complications.
- Provide chest physiotherapy as ordered.
- Give antibiotics as ordered.
- Ensure adequate fluid intake and nutrition.
- Monitor the patient's sputum and provide frequent mouth care.
- Teach prevention of community-acquired pneumonia and influenza, including appropriate vaccination.

*A*sthma

Asthma is one type of chronic obstructive pulmonary disease characterized by airflow resistance. Although asthma is a chronic reactive airway disorder, it may also present as an acute attack. Bronchospasms, increased mucus secretion, and mucosal edema cause episodic airway obstruction.

Although asthma can strike at any age, about half of all patients are younger than age 10. In this age-group, twice as many boys as girls are affected. Also, about one-third of patients contract asthma between ages 10 and 30. In this group, incidence is the same in both sexes.

About one-third of patients share the disease with at least one immediate family member.

Causes

Extrinsic, or *atopic,* asthma is a sensitivity caused by specific external allergens, such as:
- pollen
- animal dander
- house dust or mold
- kapok or feather pillows
- food additives containing sulfites.

Intrinsic, or *nonatopic,* asthma is a reaction to internal, nonallergenic factors, such as:
- severe respiratory tract infection (especially in adults)
- irritants
- emotional stress
- fatigue
- endocrine changes
- temperature and humidity variations
- exposure to noxious fumes.

Many asthmatics, especially children, have both intrinsic and extrinsic asthma.

Pathophysiology

In asthma, bronchial linings overreact to various stimuli, causing episodic smooth-muscle spasms that severely constrict the airways. Mucosal edema and thickened secretions further block the airways. (See *Understanding asthma,* pages 316 and 317.)

(Text continues on page 318.)

Understanding asthma

Asthma is an inflammatory disease characterized by hyperresponsive airways and bronchospasm. These illustrations show how an asthma attack progresses.

1. Histamine (H) attaches to receptor sites in the larger bronchi, where it causes swelling in smooth muscles.

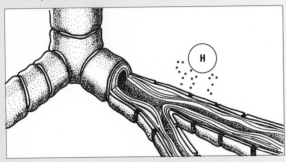

2. Slow-reacting substance of anaphylaxis (SRS-A) attaches to receptor sites in the smaller bronchi and causes swelling of smooth muscle there. SRS-A also causes fatty acids called prostaglandins to travel through the bloodstream to the lungs, where they enhance histamine effects.

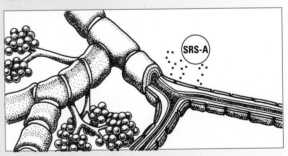

3. Histamine stimulates the mucous membranes to secrete excessive mucus, further narrowing the bronchial lumen, as shown below.

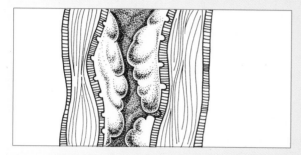

4. On inhalation, the narrowed bronchial lumen can still expand slightly, allowing air to reach the alveoli. On exhalation, increased intrathoracic pressure closes the bronchial lumen completely.

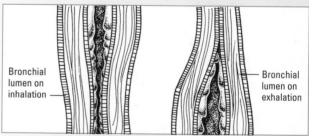

Bronchial lumen on inhalation

Bronchial lumen on exhalation

5. Mucus fills the lung bases, inhibiting alveolar ventilation. Blood, shunted to alveoli in other lung parts, still can't compensate for diminished ventilation.

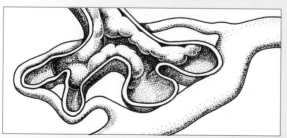

Assessment

Signs and symptoms vary depending on the severity of a patient's asthma. Patients with mild asthma have adequate air exchange and are asymptomatic between attacks. Signs and symptoms typically arise after exposure to an allergen or trigger and include:

■ brief episodes of wheezing, coughing, and dyspnea on exertion
■ intermittent episodes of wheezing, coughing, and dyspnea (typically lasting less than 1 hour, once or twice per week).

Patients with moderate asthma have normal or below-normal air exchange as well as signs and symptoms that include:

■ respiratory distress at rest
■ hyperpnea (an abnormal increase in the depth and rate of respiration)
■ exacerbations that last several days.

Patients may develop status asthmaticus, a severe attack that doesn't respond to conventional treatment. Signs and symptoms of this potentially life-threatening condition include:

■ marked respiratory distress
■ marked wheezing or absent breath sounds
■ pulsus paradoxus greater than 10 mm Hg
■ chest wall contractions.

Diagnostic tests

Pulmonary function tests (PFTs) reveal signs of airway obstructive disease, low-normal or decreased vital capacity, and increased total lung and residual capacities. Pulmonary function may be normal between attacks. PFTs are assessed before and after the patient uses a short-acting bronchodilator. Partial pressure of arterial oxygen (PaO_2) and partial pressure of arterial carbon dioxide ($PaCO_2$) are usually decreased, except in severe asthma, when $PaCO_2$ may be normal or increased, indicating severe bronchial obstruction.

Serum immunoglobulin E levels may increase from an allergic reaction. CBC with differential reveals increased eosinophil count.

Chest X-rays can diagnose or monitor asthma's progress and may show hyperinflation with areas of atelectasis. Arterial blood gas analysis detects hypoxemia and guides treatment. Pulse oximetry may show a reduced oxygen saturation level.

Skin testing may identify specific allergens. Test results are read in 1 to 2 days to detect an early reaction and again after 4 to 5 days to reveal a late reaction. Bronchial challenge testing evaluates the clinical significance of allergens identified by skin testing.

Treatment

Identifying and avoiding precipitating factors to prevent an asthma attack is the best treatment. If the stimuli can't be removed entirely, desensitization to specific antigens may be helpful. A stepwise approach may be used to control symptoms of asthma and is based on frequency and severity of symptoms along with response to medications.

Patients may need treatment with bronchodilators to decrease bronchoconstriction, reduce bronchial airway edema, and increase pulmonary ventilation. Corticosteroids have the same effects as bronchodilators; they also have anti-inflammatory and immunosuppressive effects. Mast cell stabilizers block the acute obstructive effects of antigen exposure, thereby preventing the release of the chemical mediators responsible for anaphylaxis. Leukotriene receptor antagonists are used to reduce inflammation and prevent bronchoconstriction.

If the patient is experiencing dyspnea, cyanosis, or hypoxemia, oxygen administration may be necessary. The amount delivered is designed to maintain the patient's PaO_2 between 65 and 85 mm Hg. Mechanical ventilation is needed if the patient doesn't respond to initial ventilatory support and drugs or develops respiratory failure.

Patient care

Include these measures when caring for the patient with asthma:
- Perform careful, frequent assessments of the patient's respiratory status, including respiratory rate, breath sounds, and oxygen saturation levels.
- Take action when a patient with wheezes suddenly stops wheezing and continues to show signs of respiratory distress. The absence of wheezing may be due to bronchial constriction that narrows the airways severely. So little air passes through the narrowed airways that sound is no longer produced. This is a sign of imminent respiratory collapse; the patient needs intubation and mechanical ventilation. Notify the doctor immediately and remain with the patient.
- Assess the patient's mental status for confusion, agitation, or lethargy.
- Assess the patient's heart rate and rhythm. Monitor for cardiac arrhythmias related to bronchodilator therapy or hypoxemia.
- Give drugs and I.V. fluids as ordered.
- Position the patient for maximum comfort, and provide emotional support and reassurance.

Atelectasis

Atelectasis, a condition marked by partial or total lung collapse and incomplete gas exchange, may be chronic or acute and commonly occurs to some degree in patients undergoing abdominal or thoracic surgery.

The prognosis depends on prompt removal of airway obstruction, relief of hypoxia, and reexpansion of the collapsed lobules or lung.

Causes

Atelectasis may result from:
- bronchial occlusion by mucus plugs (a common problem in heavy smokers or people with chronic obstructive pulmonary disease, bronchiectasis, or cystic fibrosis)
- occlusion by foreign bodies
- bronchogenic carcinoma
- inflammatory lung disease
- oxygen toxicity
- pulmonary edema
- any condition that inhibits full lung expansion or makes deep breathing painful, such as abdominal surgical incisions, rib fractures, tight dressings, and obesity
- prolonged immobility
- mechanical ventilation using constant small tidal volumes without intermittent deep breaths
- central nervous system depression (as in drug overdose), which eliminates periodic sighing.

Pathophysiology

In atelectasis, incomplete expansion of lobules (clusters of alveoli) or lung segments leads to partial or complete lung collapse.

Because parts of the lung are unavailable for gas exchange, unoxygenated blood passes through these areas unchanged, resulting in hypoxemia.

Assessment

Your assessment findings will vary with the cause and degree of hypoxia and may include:
- dyspnea (possibly mild and subsiding without treatment if atelectasis involves only a small area of the lung, or severe if massive collapse occurs)
- cyanosis

- decreased breath sounds
- anxiety and diaphoresis
- dull sound on percussion if a large portion of the lung is collapsed
- hypoxemia and tachycardia
- substernal or intercostal retraction
- compensatory hyperinflation of unaffected areas of the lung
- mediastinal shift to the affected side.

Diagnostic tests

Chest X-rays show characteristic horizontal lines in the lower lung zones. Dense shadows accompany segmental or lobar collapse and are commonly associated with hyperinflation of neighboring lung zones during widespread atelectasis. Extensive areas of "micro-atelectasis" may exist, however, without showing abnormalities on the patient's chest X-ray.

When the cause of atelectasis is unknown, bronchoscopy may be performed to rule out an obstructing neoplasm or a foreign body.

Treatment

Atelectasis is treated with incentive spirometry, chest percussion, postural drainage, and frequent coughing and deep-breathing exercises.

If these measures fail, bronchoscopy may help remove secretions. Humidity and bronchodilators can improve mucociliary clearance and dilate airways and are sometimes used with a nebulizer. Atelectasis secondary to an obstructing neoplasm may require surgery or radiation therapy.

Patient care

Your goal is to keep the patient's airways clear and relieve hypoxia. To achieve this, follow these guidelines:

- To prevent atelectasis, encourage the patient to cough, turn, and breathe deeply every 1 to 2 hours as ordered. Teach the patient to splint his incision when coughing. Gently reposition a postoperative patient often, and help him ambulate as soon as possible. Administer adequate analgesics to control pain.
- During mechanical ventilation, tidal volume should be maintained at 10 to 15 ml/kg of the patient's body weight to ensure adequate lung expansion. Use the sigh mechanism on the ventilator, if appropriate, to intermittently increase tidal volume at the rate of three to four sighs per hour.

Teaching the patient with atelectasis

Teach a patient with atelectasis how to use an incentive spirometer. Urge him to use it for 10 to 20 breaths every hour while he's awake. Also, teach him about respiratory care, including postural drainage, coughing, and deep breathing.

Encourage the patient to stop smoking and to lose weight if needed. Refer him to appropriate support groups for ongoing help. Because the patient may be frightened by his limited breathing capacity, provide reassurance and emotional support.

■ Humidify inspired air, and encourage adequate fluid intake to mobilize secretions. Loosen and clear secretions with postural drainage and chest percussion.
■ Assess breath sounds and ventilatory status frequently, and report changes.
■ Evaluate the patient. Secretions should be clear, and the patient should show no signs of hypoxia. (See *Teaching the patient with atelectasis*.)

Bronchiectasis

An irreversible condition marked by chronic abnormal dilation of bronchi and destruction of bronchial walls, bronchiectasis can occur throughout the tracheobronchial tree or can be confined to one segment or lobe.

However, bronchiectasis is usually bilateral, involving the basilar segments of the lower lobes. It affects people of both sexes and all ages.

Causes

Bronchiectasis may be caused by such conditions as:
■ mucoviscidosis (cystic fibrosis of the pancreas)
■ immunologic disorders such as agammaglobulinemia
■ recurrent, inadequately treated bacterial respiratory tract infections such as tuberculosis
■ measles, pneumonia, pertussis, or influenza
■ obstruction by a foreign body, tumor, or stenosis associated with recurrent infection

■ inhalation of corrosive gas or repeated aspiration of gastric juices into the lungs.

Pathophysiology

Bronchiectasis results from repeated damage to bronchial walls and abnormal mucociliary clearance that causes breakdown of supportive tissue adjacent to the airways. This disease has three forms: cylindrical (fusiform), varicose, and saccular (cystic).

Assessment

Initially, bronchiectasis may not produce symptoms. Assess your patient for a chronic cough that produces copious, foul-smelling, mucopurulent secretions, possibly totaling several cupfuls daily (classic symptom). Other characteristic findings include:

■ coarse crackles during inspiration over involved lobes or segments
■ occasional wheezes
■ dyspnea
■ weight loss and malaise
■ clubbing of fingers and toes
■ recurrent fever, chills, and other signs of infection.

Diagnostic tests

In addition to aiding diagnosis, the following tests also help determine the physiologic severity of the disease and the effects of therapy and help evaluate the patient for surgery:

■ Bronchography is the most reliable diagnostic test and reveals the location and extent of disease.
■ Chest X-rays show peribronchial thickening, areas of atelectasis, and scattered cystic changes.
■ Bronchoscopy helps identify the source of secretions or the site of bleeding in hemoptysis.
■ Sputum culture and Gram stain identify predominant organisms.
■ Complete blood count and white blood cell differential identify anemia and leukocytosis.
■ Pulmonary function tests detect decreased vital capacity and decreased expiratory flow.
■ Arterial blood gas analysis shows hypoxemia.

Treatment

Patients with bronchiectasis typically receive antibiotics by mouth or I.V. for 7 to 10 days or until sputum production decreases. If the pa-

Teaching the patient with bronchiectasis

When caring for a patient with bronchiectasis, make sure to explain all diagnostic tests. Urge the patient to stop smoking because it stimulates secretions and irritates the airways, and refer him to a local self-help group.

Show family members how to perform postural drainage and percussion. Also, teach the patient coughing and deep-breathing techniques to promote ventilation and removal of secretions. Teach the patient how to dispose of secretions properly.

Caution the patient to avoid air pollutants and people with upper respiratory tract infections. Instruct him to take medications (especially antibiotics) exactly as prescribed. To help prevent this disease, vigorously treat bacterial pneumonia, and stress the need for immunization to prevent childhood diseases.

tient has bronchospasm and thick, tenacious sputum, bronchodilators may be given along with postural drainage and chest percussion to help remove secretions. Occasionally, bronchoscopy may be used to aid removal of secretions.

The patient may also need oxygen therapy to treat hypoxemia. If hemoptysis is severe, lobectomy or segmental resection may be performed.

Patient care

Care is mainly supportive. Incorporate the following measures into a care plan:
■ Provide a warm, quiet, comfortable environment, and urge the patient to rest as much as possible.
■ Administer antibiotics as ordered.
■ Perform chest physiotherapy several times per day (early morning and bedtime are best); include postural drainage and chest percussion for involved lobes. Have the patient maintain each position for 10 minutes; then perform percussion and instruct him to cough.
■ Encourage balanced, high-protein meals to promote good health and tissue healing and plenty of fluids to aid expectoration.
■ Provide frequent mouth care to remove foul-smelling sputum.
■ Evaluate the patient. His secretions should be thin and clear or white. (See *Teaching the patient with bronchiectasis*.)

Chronic obstructive pulmonary disease

Chronic obstructive pulmonary disease (COPD) is an umbrella term that may refer to emphysema, chronic bronchitis, asthma and, more commonly, any combination of these conditions (usually bronchitis and emphysema). The most common chronic lung disease, COPD affects an estimated 30 million Americans, and its incidence is rising. It now ranks third among the major causes of death in the United States.

COPD affects more men than women, probably because until recently men were more likely to smoke heavily. However, the rate of COPD among women is increasing. Early COPD may not produce symptoms and may cause only minimal disability in many patients, but it tends to worsen with time.

Causes

COPD may be caused by:
- cigarette smoking
- recurrent or chronic respiratory tract infection
- allergies
- familial and hereditary factors such as alpha$_1$-antitrypsin deficiency.

Pathophysiology

Smoking, one of the major causes of COPD, impairs ciliary action and macrophage function and causes inflammation in the airways, increased mucus production, destruction of alveolar septa, and peribronchiolar fibrosis. Early inflammatory changes may reverse if the patient stops smoking before lung disease becomes extensive.

The mucus plugs and narrowed airways cause air trapping, as in chronic bronchitis and emphysema. Hyperinflation of the alveoli occurs on expiration. On inspiration, airways enlarge, allowing air to pass beyond the obstruction; on expiration, airways narrow, preventing gas flow. Air trapping (also called *ball valving*) occurs commonly in asthma and chronic bronchitis.

Assessment

The typical patient with COPD is asymptomatic until middle age, when the following signs and symptoms may occur:
- reduced ability to exercise or do strenuous work
- productive cough
- dyspnea with minimal exertion
- diminished, low-pitched breath sounds

<u>**Teaching the patient with COPD**</u>

If your patient has chronic obstructive pulmonary disease (COPD), familiarize him with prescribed bronchodilators. Explain that they alleviate bronchospasm and improve mucociliary clearance of secretions. Teach or reinforce the correct way to use an inhaler.

To strengthen respiratory muscles, teach the patient to take slow, deep breaths and to exhale through pursed lips. Teach him how to cough effectively to help mobilize secretions. If secretions are thick, urge the patient to drink 12 to 15 glasses of fluid daily.

Urge the patient to stop smoking and to avoid other respiratory irritants. Mention that an air conditioner with an air filter may prove helpful. If the patient will continue oxygen therapy at home, teach him how to use the equipment correctly.

- sonorous or sibilant wheezes (or both)
- prolonged expiration
- fine, inspiratory crackles.

Diagnostic tests

In advanced disease, a chest X-ray reveals a flattened diaphragm, reduced vascular markings at the lung periphery, hyperinflation of the lungs, a vertical heart, enlarged anteroposterior chest diameter, and a large retrosternal air space. Pulmonary function tests show increased residual volume, total lung capacity, and compliance as well as decreased vital capacity, diffusing capacity, and expiratory volumes. Arterial blood gas (ABG) analysis indicates a reduced partial pressure of arterial oxygen (PaO_2) with normal partial pressure of arterial carbon dioxide until late in the disease.

At later stages, electrocardiography will reveal signs of right ventricular hypertrophy, such as tall, symmetrical P waves in leads II, III, and aV_F; and vertical QRS axis. Late in the disease when persistent severe hypoxia is present, a red blood cell count will show increased hemoglobin levels.

Treatment

Treatment for COPD aims to relieve symptoms and prevent complications. Most patients receive beta-adrenergic agonist bronchodilators (albuterol or salmeterol), anticholinergic bronchodilators (ipratropium), and corticosteroids (beclomethasone or triamcinolone). These drugs are usually given by metered-dose inhaler. Lung-volume reduction surgery improves exercise capacity and quality of life in some patients with severe emphysema.

Patient care

Your care should include these measures:
- Give antibiotics, as ordered, to treat respiratory tract infections.
- Give low concentrations of oxygen as ordered.
- Check ABG values regularly to determine oxygen need and to avoid carbon dioxide narcosis.
- Evaluate the patient. The patient's chest X-rays, respiratory rate and rhythm, ABG values, and pH should be normal. PaO_2 should be greater than 60 mm Hg. Body weight and urine output should also be normal. (See *Teaching the patient with COPD.*)

Cor pulmonale

In cor pulmonale, or right ventricular hypertrophy, the ventricle enlarges and dilates at the end stage of a disease that affects the structure, function, or vasculature of the lungs, in some cases resulting in heart failure. It doesn't occur, however, with disorders stemming from congenital heart disease or those affecting the left side of the heart.

About 85% of patients with cor pulmonale also have chronic obstructive pulmonary disease (COPD), and about 25% of patients with bronchial COPD eventually develop cor pulmonale. It's most common in smokers and in middle-aged and elderly men; however, the incidence in women is rising.

Causes

Cor pulmonale may result from:
- disorders that affect the pulmonary parenchyma
- pulmonary diseases that affect the airways (such as COPD and bronchial asthma)
- vascular diseases (such as vasculitis, pulmonary emboli, or external vascular obstruction from a tumor or aneurysm)
- chest wall abnormalities (such as kyphoscoliosis and pectus excavatum [funnel chest])
- neuromuscular disorders (such as muscular dystrophy and poliomyelitis)
- external factors (such as obesity or living at a high altitude).

Pathophysiology

In cor pulmonale, pulmonary hypertension increases the heart's workload. To compensate, the right ventricle hypertrophies to force blood through the lungs. As long as the heart can compensate for the increased pulmonary vascular resistance, signs and symptoms reflect only the underlying disorder.

Assessment

In early stages of cor pulmonale, patients are most likely to report:
- chronic productive cough
- exertional dyspnea
- wheezing respirations
- fatigue and weakness.

As the compensatory mechanism begins to fail, larger amounts of blood remain in the right ventricle at the end of diastole, causing ventricular dilation. As cor pulmonale progresses, these additional symptoms occur:
- dyspnea at rest
- tachypnea
- orthopnea
- dependent edema
- jugular vein distention
- enlarged, tender liver
- hepatojugular reflux (jugular vein distention induced by pressing over the liver)
- right upper quadrant discomfort
- tachycardia
- systolic ejection murmur
- decreased cardiac output.

Chest examination reveals characteristics of the underlying lung disease.

In response to hypoxia, the bone marrow produces more red blood cells (RBCs), causing polycythemia. The blood's viscosity increases, which further aggravates pulmonary hypertension. This increases the right ventricle's workload, causing heart failure.

Eventually, cor pulmonale may lead to biventricular failure, hepatomegaly, edema, ascites, and pleural effusions. Polycythemia increases the risk of thromboembolism. Because cor pulmonale occurs late in the course of COPD and other irreversible diseases, the prognosis is poor. (See *Understanding cor pulmonale.*)

Understanding cor pulmonale

Three types of disorders are responsible for cor pulmonale:
- pulmonary restrictive disorders, such as fibrosis or obesity
- pulmonary obstructive disorders, such as bronchitis
- primary vascular disorders, such as recurrent pulmonary emboli.

   These disorders share a common pathway to the formation of cor pulmonale, as shown in this flowchart. Hypoxic constriction of pulmonary blood vessels and obstruction of pulmonary blood flow lead to increased pulmonary resistance, which progresses to cor pulmonale.

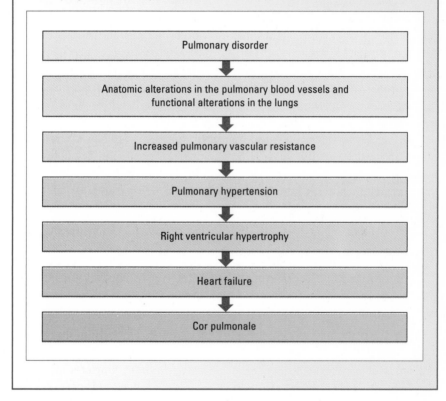

Pulmonary disorder

⬇

Anatomic alterations in the pulmonary blood vessels and functional alterations in the lungs

⬇

Increased pulmonary vascular resistance

⬇

Pulmonary hypertension

⬇

Right ventricular hypertrophy

⬇

Heart failure

⬇

Cor pulmonale

Diagnostic tests

The following tests are used to diagnose cor pulmonale:
- Pulmonary artery (PA) catheterization shows increased right ventricular and PA pressures, resulting from increased pulmonary vascular resistance. Both right ventricular systolic and PA systolic pressures are above 30 mm Hg, and PA diastolic pressure is higher than 15 mm Hg.

- Echocardiography or angiography demonstrates right ventricular enlargement.
- Chest X-rays reveal large central pulmonary arteries and right ventricular enlargement.
- Arterial blood gas analysis detects decreased partial pressure of arterial oxygen (usually less than 70 mm Hg and never more than 90 mm Hg).
- Ventilation-perfusion scan may be performed if pulmonary embolus is the suspected cause.
- Pulse oximetry shows a reduced oxygen saturation level.
- Electrocardiography discloses arrhythmias, such as premature atrial and ventricular contractions and atrial fibrillation during severe hypoxia. It may also show right bundle-branch block, right axis deviation, prominent P waves, and an inverted T wave in right precordial leads.
- Pulmonary function tests reflect underlying pulmonary disease.
- Magnetic resonance imaging measures right ventricular mass, wall thickness, and ejection fraction.
- Cardiac catheterization measures pulmonary vascular pressures.
- Hematocrit typically exceeds 50%.
- Serum liver enzyme levels show an elevated level of aspartate aminotransferase with hepatic congestion and decreased liver function.
- Serum bilirubin levels may be elevated if liver dysfunction and hepatomegaly are present.

Treatment

Treatment for cor pulmonale aims to reduce hypoxemia and pulmonary vasoconstriction, increase exercise tolerance, and correct underlying conditions. Treatment measures include bed rest, antibiotics for respiratory infections, diuretics, pulmonary artery vasodilators, and continuous administration of low concentrations of oxygen. Patients should also receive a low-sodium diet and restricted fluids.

Phlebotomy, to decrease RBC mass if hematocrit exceeds 65%, along with anticoagulation using small doses of warfarin or heparin, may decrease the risk of thromboembolism. In cases of acute disease, the patient may require mechanical ventilation.

Patient care

When caring for a patient with cor pulmonale, follow these steps:
- Make sure that the patient receives a low-sodium diet.
- Monitor the patient's fluid intake.

- Give antibiotics and vasodilators as ordered.
- Give oxygen as ordered.
- Monitor the patient's respiratory status.

Pleural effusion

Pleural effusion is an excess of fluid in the pleural space. Normally, this space contains a small amount of extracellular fluid that lubricates the pleural surfaces. Increased production or inadequate removal of this fluid results in transudative or exudative pleural effusion. Empyema, the accumulation of pus and necrotic tissue in the pleural space, is also a form of pleural effusion.

Causes

Transudative pleural effusion can stem from:
- heart failure
- hepatic disease with ascites
- peritoneal dialysis
- hypoalbuminemia
- disorders resulting in overexpanded intravascular volume.
  Exudative pleural effusion can stem from:
- tuberculosis (TB)
- subphrenic abscess
- esophageal rupture
- pancreatitis
- bacterial or fungal pneumonitis
- empyema
- cancer
- pulmonary embolism with or without infarction
- collagen disorders (such as lupus erythematosus and rheumatoid arthritis)
- myxedema
- chest trauma.

Pathophysiology

In transudative pleural effusion, excessive hydrostatic pressure or decreased osmotic pressure allows excessive fluid to pass across intact capillaries, resulting in an ultrafiltrate of plasma containing low concentrations of protein.

In exudative pleural effusion, capillaries exhibit increased permeability, with or without changes in hydrostatic and colloid osmotic pressures, allowing protein-rich fluid to leak into the pleural space. Empyema is usually associated with infection in the pleural space.

Assessment

Assess your patient for these signs and symptoms:
- dyspnea
- dry cough
- pleural friction rub
- possible pleuritic pain that worsens with coughing or deep breathing
- dullness on percussion
- tachycardia
- tachypnea
- decreased chest motion and breath sounds
- mediastinal shift with large effusion.

Diagnostic tests

Examination of pleural fluid obtained by thoracentesis reveals these findings:
- In transudative effusions, specific gravity is usually less than 1.015 and protein less than 3 g/dl.
- In exudative effusions, specific gravity is greater than 1.02, and the ratio of protein in pleural fluid to serum is equal to or greater than 0.5. Pleural fluid lactate dehydrogenase (LD) is equal to or greater than 200 IU, and the ratio of LD in pleural fluid to LD in serum is equal to or greater than 0.6.
- If a pleural effusion results from esophageal rupture or pancreatitis, amylase levels in aspirated fluid are usually higher than serum levels.
- In empyema, cell analysis shows leukocytosis.
- Aspirated fluid may also be tested for lupus erythematosus cells, antinuclear antibodies, and neoplastic cells. It may be analyzed for color and consistency; acid-fast bacillus, fungal, and bacterial cultures; and triglycerides (in chylothorax).
- Chest X-ray shows radiopaque fluid in dependent regions.
- Pleural biopsy may be particularly useful for confirming tuberculosis or cancer.

Treatment

Depending on the amount of fluid present, symptomatic effusion requires either thoracentesis to remove fluid or careful monitoring of the

Teaching the patient with pleural effusion

If your patient has pleural effusion, teach him what to expect in a thoracentesis. Reassure him during the procedure, and watch for complications.

Encourage the patient to perform deep-breathing exercises to promote lung expansion and to use an incentive spirometer to promote deep breathing.

patient's own fluid reabsorption. Hemothorax requires drainage to prevent fibrothorax formation. Associated hypoxia requires supplemental oxygen.

Patient care

Implement these measures as part of your care:

- Administer oxygen as ordered.
- Provide meticulous chest tube care, and use sterile technique for changing dressings around the tube insertion site in empyema. Record the amount, color, and consistency of tube drainage.
- If the patient has open drainage through a rib resection or an intercostal tube, follow standard precautions. Because weeks of such drainage are usually necessary to obliterate the space, make visiting nurse referrals for patients who will be discharged with the tube in place.
- If pleural effusion was a complication of pneumonia or influenza, advise the patient to seek prompt medical attention for chest colds.
- Evaluate the patient. He should remain afebrile and have minimal chest discomfort and a normal respiratory pattern. (See *Teaching the patient with pleural effusion.*)

Pneumonia

Pneumonia is an acute infection of the lung parenchyma that commonly impairs gas exchange. The prognosis is usually good for people who have normal lungs and adequate host defenses before the onset of pneumonia; however, bacterial pneumonia is the fifth leading cause of death in debilitated patients. The disorder occurs in primary and secondary forms.

Causes

Pneumonia is caused by an infecting pathogen (bacterial or viral) or by a chemical or other irritant (such as aspirated material). Certain predisposing factors increase the risk of pneumonia.

For bacterial and viral pneumonia, these include:
- chronic illness and debilitation
- cancer (particularly lung cancer)
- abdominal and thoracic surgery
- atelectasis
- aspiration
- colds or other viral respiratory infections
- chronic respiratory disease, such as chronic obstructive pulmonary disease (COPD), asthma, bronchiectasis, and cystic fibrosis
- smoking, alcoholism
- malnutrition
- sickle cell disease
- tracheostomy
- exposure to noxious gases
- immunosuppressive therapy.

Aspiration pneumonia is more likely to occur in elderly or debilitated patients, those receiving nasogastric (NG) tube feedings, and those with an impaired gag reflex, poor oral hygiene, or a decreased level of consciousness.

 AGE ALERT Older adults are at greater risk for developing pneumonia because their weakened chest muscles reduce their ability to clear secretions. Those in long-term care facilities are especially susceptible.

Bacterial pneumonia is the most common type found in older adults; viral pneumonia is the second most common type. Aspiration pneumonia results from impaired swallowing ability and a diminished gag reflex due to stroke or prolonged illness.

An older adult with pneumonia may have fatigue, a slight cough, and a rapid respiratory rate. Pleuritic pain and fever may be present. Keep in mind that an absence of fever doesn't mean absence of infection in an older adult. Many older adults develop a subnormal body temperature in response to infection.

Pathophysiology

In general, the lower respiratory tract can be exposed to pathogens by inhalation, aspiration, vascular dissemination, or direct contact with contaminated equipment such as suction catheters. After pathogens are inside, they begin to colonize and infection develops.

In bacterial pneumonia, which can occur in any part of the lungs, an infection initially triggers alveolar inflammation and edema. This produces an area of low ventilation with normal perfusion. Capillaries become engorged with blood, causing stasis. As the alveolar capillary membrane breaks down, alveoli fill with blood and exudate, resulting in atelectasis. In severe bacterial infections, the lungs look heavy and liverlike—similar to acute respiratory distress syndrome.

In viral pneumonia, the virus first attacks bronchiolar epithelial cells. This causes interstitial inflammation and desquamation. The virus also invades bronchial mucous glands and goblet cells. It then spreads to the alveoli, which fill with blood and fluid.

In aspiration pneumonia, inhalation of gastric juices or hydrocarbons triggers inflammatory changes and inactivates surfactant over a large area. Decreased surfactant leads to alveolar collapse. Acidic gastric juices may damage the airways and alveoli. Particles containing aspirated gastric juices may obstruct the airways and reduce airflow, leading to secondary bacterial pneumonia.

Assessment

The five cardinal signs and symptoms of early bacterial pneumonia are:
- coughing
- sputum production
- pleuritic chest pain
- shaking chills
- fever.

Other signs vary widely, ranging from diffuse, fine crackles to signs of localized or extensive consolidation and pleural effusion.

Diagnostic tests

Chest X-rays showing infiltrates and a sputum smear demonstrating acute inflammatory cells support the diagnosis. Positive blood cultures in patients with pulmonary infiltrates strongly suggest pneumonia produced by the organisms isolated from the blood cultures.

Occasionally, a transtracheal aspirate of tracheobronchial secretions or bronchoscopy with brushings may be performed to obtain material for smear and culture. Early *Pneumocystis jiroveci* (formerly *carinii*) pneumonia can be detected only by a ventilation-perfusion scan.

Treatment

Antimicrobial therapy varies with the infecting agent. Therapy should be reevaluated early in the course of treatment.

Teaching the patient with pneumonia

Teach the patient how to cough and perform deep-breathing exercises to clear secretions. In addition, teach the patient how to prevent later bouts of pneumonia.

For example, urge all postoperative and bedridden patients to perform deep-breathing exercises often. Position patients properly to promote full ventilation and drainage of secretions.

Also encourage annual influenza and pneumococcal vaccination for high-risk patients, such as those with chronic obstructive pulmonary disease, chronic heart disease, or sickle cell disease.

Furthermore, advise patients to avoid indiscriminate antibiotic use during minor viral infections. Explain that doing so may promote colonization of antibiotic-resistant bacteria in the upper airways. If the patient then develops pneumonia, the infecting organisms may need treatment with more toxic antibiotics.

Supportive measures include humidified oxygen therapy for hypoxemia, mechanical ventilation for respiratory failure, a high-calorie diet and adequate fluid intake, and bed rest. Patients may receive an analgesic to relieve pleuritic chest pain.

Patient care

These interventions aim to increase patient comfort, avoid complications, and speed recovery:

- Maintain a patent airway and adequate oxygenation. Measure arterial blood gas (ABG) levels, especially in hypoxic patients. Administer supplemental oxygen as ordered. Use caution when administering oxygen to patients with underlying COPD.
- Give antibiotics as ordered and pain medication as needed. Fever and dehydration may warrant I.V. fluids and electrolyte replacement.
- Maintain adequate nutrition to offset extra calories burned during infection. Ask the dietary department to provide a high-calorie, high-protein diet consisting of soft, easy-to-eat foods. Encourage the patient to eat. Monitor fluid intake and output.
- To control the spread of infection, dispose of secretions properly. Tell the patient to sneeze and cough into a disposable tissue; tape a waxed bag to the side of the bed for used tissues.
- To prevent aspiration during NG tube feedings, elevate the patient's head, check the position of the tube, and administer feedings slowly. Don't give large volumes at one time because this could cause vomit-

ing. If the patient has a tracheostomy or an endotracheal tube, inflate the tube cuff. Keep his head elevated for at least 30 minutes after feeding.

■ Be aware that antimicrobial agents used to treat cytomegalovirus, *P. jiroveci,* and respiratory syncytial virus pneumonia may be hazardous to fetal development. Pregnant health care workers or those attempting conception should minimize exposure to these agents (such as acyclovir [Zovirax], ribavirin [Virazole], and pentamidine [NebuPent]).

■ Evaluate the patient. His chest X-rays should be normal and his ABG levels should show partial pressure of arterial oxygen of 50 to 60 mm Hg. (See *Teaching the patient with pneumonia.*)

Pneumothorax

In pneumothorax, air or gas accumulates between the parietal and visceral pleurae, causing the lungs to collapse. The amount of air or gas trapped determines the degree of lung collapse. In some cases, venous return to the heart is impeded, causing a life-threatening condition called *tension pneumothorax.*

Pneumothorax is classified as either traumatic or spontaneous. Traumatic pneumothorax may be further classified as open (sucking chest wound) or closed (blunt or penetrating trauma). Note that if an open (penetrating) wound seals itself off, stopping communication between the atmosphere and the pleural space, a closed pneumothorax may result. Spontaneous pneumothorax, which is also considered closed, can be further classified as *primary* (idiopathic) or *secondary* (related to a specific disease).

Causes

Traumatic pneumothorax can result from:
■ insertion of a central venous pressure line
■ thoracic surgery
■ thoracentesis or closed pleural biopsy
■ penetrating chest injury
■ transbronchial biopsy.

Spontaneous pneumothorax can result from:
■ ruptured congenital blebs
■ ruptured emphysematous bullae
■ tubercular or malignant lesions that erode into the pleural space
■ interstitial lung disease such as eosinophilic granuloma.

Understanding tension pneumothorax

In tension pneumothorax, air accumulates intrapleurally and can't escape. Intrapleural pressure rises, collapsing the ipsilateral lung.

Breathing in
With inspiration, the mediastinum shifts toward the unaffected lung, impairing ventilation.

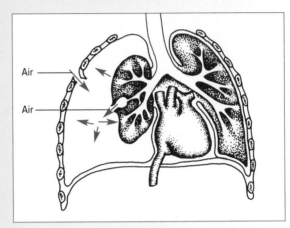

Air

Air

Breathing out
With expiration, the mediastinal shift distorts the vena cava and reduces venous return.

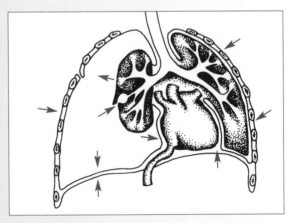

Tension pneumothorax can develop from either traumatic or spontaneous pneumothorax. (See *Understanding tension pneumothorax.*)

Pathophysiology

The pathophysiology of pneumothorax varies according to classification. Open pneumothorax results when atmospheric air (positive pressure) flows directly into the pleural cavity (negative pressure). As the air pressure in the pleural cavity becomes positive, the lung collapses on the affected side. Lung collapse leads to decreased total lung capacity, causing hypoxia.

Closed pneumothorax occurs when air enters the pleural space from within the lung. This causes increased pleural pressure, which prevents lung expansion during inspiration. It may be called traumatic pneumothorax when blunt chest trauma causes lung tissue to rupture, resulting in air leakage.

Spontaneous pneumothorax is a type of closed pneumothorax that usually results when a subpleural bleb (a small cystic space) at the surface of the lung ruptures. This rupture causes air leakage into the pleural spaces; then the lung collapses, causing decreased total lung capacity, vital capacity, and lung compliance—leading, in turn, to hypoxia.

Assessment

Spontaneous pneumothorax may not produce symptoms in mild cases, but profound respiratory distress occurs in moderate to severe cases. Weak and rapid pulse, pallor, jugular vein distention, and anxiety indicate tension pneumothorax. In most cases, look for these symptoms:
- sudden, sharp, pleuritic pain
- asymmetrical chest wall movement
- shortness of breath
- cyanosis
- decreased or absent breath sounds over the collapsed lung
- hyperresonance on the affected side
- crackling beneath the skin on palpation (subcutaneous emphysema).

Diagnostic tests

- Chest X-rays show air in the pleural space and may reveal mediastinal shift.
- If pneumothorax is significant, arterial blood gas findings include pH less than 7.35, partial pressure of arterial oxygen less than 80 mm Hg, and partial pressure of arterial carbon dioxide above 45 mm Hg.

Treatment

Treatment is conservative for spontaneous pneumothorax in cases where no signs of increased pleural pressure appear, lung collapse is less than 30%, and the patient shows no signs of dyspnea or other indications of physiologic compromise. Such treatment consists of bed rest or activity as tolerated by the patient; careful monitoring of blood pressure, pulse rate, and respirations; and oxygen administration. Some patients may require needle aspiration of the air using a large-bore needle attached to a syringe.

Keep in mind that, when more than 30% of the lung has collapsed, the patient will require a thoracotomy tube to allow air to rise to the top of the intrapleural space. Placed in the second or third intercostal space at the midclavicular line, the tube is then connected to an underwater seal with suction at low pressures.

Patients experiencing recurrent spontaneous pneumothoraxes will require a thoracotomy and pleurectomy. These procedures prevent recurrence by causing the lung to adhere to the parietal pleura. Patients with traumatic or tension pneumothorax require chest tube drainage. Traumatic pneumothorax may also require surgical repair.

Patient care

These measures aim to prevent complications and increase patient comfort:
- Watch for pallor, gasping respirations, and sudden chest pain.
- Carefully monitor vital signs at least every hour for indications of shock, increasing respiratory distress, or mediastinal shift. Listen for breath sounds over both lungs. Falling blood pressure with rising pulse and respiratory rates may indicate tension pneumothorax, which can be fatal if not promptly treated.
- Make the patient as comfortable as possible—a patient with pneumothorax is usually most comfortable sitting upright.
- Urge the patient to control coughing and gasping during thoracotomy.
- After the chest tube is in place, encourage him to cough and breathe deeply at least once per hour to facilitate lung expansion.
- In the patient undergoing chest tube drainage, watch for continuing air leakage (bubbling) in the water-seal chamber. This indicates the lung defect has failed to close and may require surgery. Also observe for increasing subcutaneous emphysema by checking around the neck or at the tube insertion site for crackling beneath the skin. If the patient is on a ventilator, be alert for difficulty in breathing in time with the ventilator as you monitor its gauges for pressure increases.
- Change dressings around the chest tube insertion site as needed and as per your facility's policy. Be careful not to reposition or dislodge the tube. If the tube dislodges, immediately place a petroleum gauze dressing over the opening to prevent rapid lung collapse.
- Observe the chest tube site for leakage, and note the amount and color of drainage. Ambulate the patient as ordered (usually on the first postoperative day) to facilitate deep inspiration and lung expansion.

Teaching the patient with pneumothorax

If your patient has pneumothorax, reassure him by explaining what occurs in pneumothorax, what causes it, and all needed diagnostic tests and procedures. Encourage the patient to perform hourly deep-breathing exercises while awake.

Discuss the possibility of recurrent spontaneous pneumothorax, and review its signs and symptoms. Stress the need for immediate medical intervention if it occurs.

■ Evaluate the patient. Chest X-rays, respiratory rate and depth, and vital signs should be normal. (See *Teaching the patient with pneumothorax*.)

Pulmonary edema

Pulmonary edema is a common complication of cardiac disorders. It's marked by accumulated fluid in the lung's extravascular spaces. It may occur as a chronic condition or develop quickly, rapidly becoming fatal.

Causes

Pulmonary edema may result from left-sided heart failure caused by:
■ arteriosclerosis
■ cardiomyopathy
■ hypertension
■ valvular heart disease.

Pathophysiology

Normally, pulmonary capillary hydrostatic pressure, capillary oncotic pressure, capillary permeability, and lymphatic drainage are in balance. This prevents fluid infiltration to the lungs. When this balance changes, or the lymphatic drainage system is obstructed, pulmonary edema results.

If colloid osmotic pressure decreases, the hydrostatic force that regulates intravascular fluids is lost because nothing opposes it. Fluid flows freely into the interstitium and alveoli, impairing gas exchange and leading to pulmonary edema. (See *Understanding pulmonary edema*, page 342.)

Understanding pulmonary edema

In pulmonary edema, reduced function in the left ventricle causes blood to pool there and in the left atrium. Eventually, blood backs up into the pulmonary veins and capillaries.

Increasing capillary hydrostatic pressure pushes fluid into the interstitial spaces and alveoli. The illustrations below show a normal alveolus and the effects of pulmonary edema.

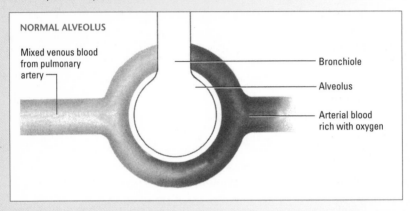

NORMAL ALVEOLUS

Mixed venous blood from pulmonary artery

Bronchiole

Alveolus

Arterial blood rich with oxygen

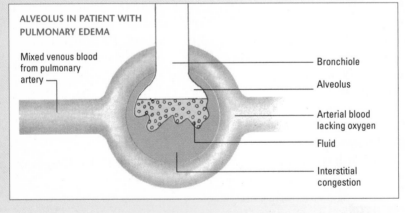

ALVEOLUS IN PATIENT WITH PULMONARY EDEMA

Mixed venous blood from pulmonary artery

Bronchiole

Alveolus

Arterial blood lacking oxygen

Fluid

Interstitial congestion

Assessment

Signs and symptoms vary with the stage of pulmonary edema. In the early stages, look for:

- dyspnea on exertion
- paroxysmal nocturnal dyspnea
- orthopnea
- cough

- mild tachypnea
- dependent crackles
- increased blood pressure
- jugular vein distention
- diastolic S_3 gallop
- tachycardia.
  As tissue hypoxia and decreased cardiac output occur, you'll see:
- labored, rapid respiration
- more diffuse crackles
- cough producing frothy, bloody sputum
- increased tachycardia
- falling blood pressure
- thready pulse
- arrhythmias
- cold, clammy skin
- diaphoresis
- cyanosis.

Diagnostic tests

Clinical features of pulmonary edema permit a working diagnosis. These diagnostic tests are used to confirm the disease:
- Arterial blood gas (ABG) analysis usually shows hypoxia with variable partial pressure of arterial carbon dioxide, depending on the patient's degree of fatigue. Metabolic acidosis may be revealed.
- Chest X-rays show diffuse haziness of the lung fields and, usually, cardiomegaly and pleural effusion. Sequential chest X-rays show whether thoracostomy was effective in resolving pneumothorax.
- Pulse oximetry may reveal decreasing oxygen saturation levels.
- Pulmonary artery (PA) catheterization identifies left-sided heart failure and helps rule out acute respiratory distress syndrome.
- Electrocardiography may show previous or current myocardial infarction.

Treatment

Treatment of pulmonary edema is directed toward reducing extravascular fluid, improving gas exchange and myocardial function, and correcting the underlying disease if possible. Patients typically receive a high concentration of oxygen delivered by cannula. If arterial oxygen levels remain low, assisted ventilation may be necessary.

Diuretics are given to mobilize extravascular fluid. Patients may also receive positive inotropic agents to enhance myocardial contractility, pressor agents to enhance contractility and promote vasoconstriction,

CASE CLIP

Responding to acute pulmonary edema

Mr. M. is a 70-year-old man with a history of heart failure and coronary artery disease. He had an aortic valve replacement 3 days earlier. His surgery was uneventful, and he was transferred out of the intensive care unit (ICU) 1 day after surgery. Mr. M.'s hemoglobin level was 7 g/dl and his hematocrit was 21%; his surgeon ordered 2 units of packed red blood cells (PRBCs), with 20 mg of I.V. furosemide to be given between units. Mr. M.'s intake and output for the previous 16 hours was balanced at 1,200 ml.

After the first unit of PRBCs was transfused, the nurse returned to assess Mr. M. and administer the furosemide. On assessment, Mr. M was experiencing dyspnea with an oxygen saturation of 87%. Telemetry showed slightly irregular sinus tachycardia at a rate of 140 beats/minute and slightly irregular. (*Note:* At a rate of 140 beats/minute, it's difficult to see PACs on a bedside monitor.) Mr. M.'s other vital signs were:
■ temperature: 102.3° F (39.1° C)
■ respiratory rate (RR): 36 breaths/minute
■ blood pressure: 90/58 mm Hg.

Mr. M. had a normal S_1/S_2, tachycardia, no jugular vein distention, and diffuse crackles in all lung fields.

The nurse called the rapid response team (RRT). While waiting for the RRT, the nurse applied a 100% non-rebreather mask and requested an immediate portable chest X-ray. The RRT respiratory therapist drew an arterial blood gas (ABG) sample and sent it out for immediate analysis. The RRT physician supported the nurse's decision for the chest X-ray and requested that a second I.V. line be started. Repeat assessment of Mr. M.

showed no improvement with oxygen therapy. Mr. M.'s vital signs were now:
■ heart rate: unchanged at 140 beats/minute
■ RR: remained 36 breaths/minute
■ pulse oximetry: 90%.

The physician discussed with Mr. M. the need for intubation and ventilator support. The responding critical care nurse notified the ICU of the transfer. The X-ray showed bilateral infiltrates that were patchy and alveolar, with a normal cardiac silhouette and no effusions. The ABG results were reported as pH 7.35, $PaCO_2$ 31 mm Hg, PaO_2 60 mm Hg and HCO_3^- 26 mEq/L. Additional laboratory tests requested by the RRT physician included brain natriuretic peptide.

The bedside nurse notified the blood bank that a transfusion reaction was suspected and arranged for the blood bag and tubing to be returned to the laboratory. Mr. M. was transferred back to the ICU, where he was urgently reintubated. The respiratory therapist documented that he had elevated peak airway pressures and frothy, pink sputum coming from his endotracheal tube. Mr. M. received continued supportive care and, 48 hours later, was well enough to be extubated and returned to the telemetry unit. The blood bank reported that the compared donor and recipient sera had identified high granulocyte counts and lymphocytotoxic antibodies. That finding supported the diagnosis of transfusion-related acute lung injury.

Within 4 days, Mr. M.'s chest X-ray had cleared. Eleven days after his surgery, Mr. M. was discharged home to complete his recovery.

and arterial vasodilators. Morphine is used to reduce anxiety and dyspnea. (See *Responding to acute pulmonary edema*.)

Patient care

When caring for a patient with pulmonary edema, consider these interventions:

■ Help the patient relax to promote oxygenation, control bronchospasm, and enhance myocardial contractility.

■ Reassure the patient, who's likely to be frightened by his inability to breathe normally. Provide emotional support to family members as well.

■ Place the patient in high Fowler's position to enhance lung expansion.

■ Administer oxygen as ordered.

■ Assess the patient's condition often, and document his responses to treatment. Monitor ABG and pulse oximetry values, oral and I.V. fluid intake, urine output and, in the patient with a PA catheter, pulmonary end-diastolic and pulmonary artery wedge pressures. Check the cardiac monitor often, and report changes immediately.

■ Watch for complications of such treatments as electrolyte depletion, oxygen therapy, and mechanical ventilation.

■ Monitor vital signs every 15 to 30 minutes while administering nitroprusside (Nitropres) in dextrose 5% in water by I.V. drip. During use, protect the solution from light by wrapping the bottle or bag with aluminum foil. Discard unused nitroprusside solution after 4 hours. Watch for arrhythmias in a patient receiving digoxin (Lanoxin), and for marked respiratory depression in a patient receiving morphine.

■ Carefully record the time morphine is given and the amount administered.

Pulmonary embolism and infarction

Pulmonary embolism is an obstruction of the pulmonary arterial bed by a dislodged thrombus or foreign substance. Pulmonary infarction, or lung tissue death from a pulmonary embolus, is sometimes mild and may not produce symptoms. However, when a massive embolism obstructs more than 50% of the pulmonary arterial circulation, it can be rapidly fatal.

Causes

Pulmonary embolism usually results from dislodged thrombi that originate in the leg veins. Other less common sources of thrombi include:

- pelvic veins
- renal veins
- hepatic vein
- right side of the heart
- arms.

Pathophysiology

Trauma, clot dissolution, sudden muscle spasm, intravascular pressure changes, or a change in peripheral blood flow can cause the thrombus to loosen or fragmentize.

The thrombus—now called an embolus—floats to the heart's right side and enters the lung through the pulmonary artery. There, the embolus may dissolve, continue to fragmentize, or grow. If the embolus occludes the pulmonary artery, alveoli collapse and atelectasis develops. If the embolus enlarges, it may clog most or all of the pulmonary vessels and cause death.

In rare cases, the emboli contain air, fat, amniotic fluid, tumor cells, or talc (sometimes found in oral drugs that are injected I.V. by addicts). (See *Responding to air or amniotic fluid embolism*.) Pulmonary embolism may lead to pulmonary infarction, especially in patients with chronic heart or pulmonary disease.

Assessment

Total occlusion of the main pulmonary artery is rapidly fatal; smaller or fragmented emboli produce symptoms that vary with the size, number, and location of the emboli. A patient with a pulmonary embolus may also be asymptomatic.

Common symptoms include:
- tachypnea
- dyspnea (usually the first symptom)
- crackles or wheezes
- anginal or pleuritic chest pain
- productive cough (sputum may be blood-tinged)
- tachycardia
- low-grade fever.
  Less common symptoms include:
- massive hemoptysis
- splinting of the chest
- leg edema.
  A large embolus may produce:
- crackles and a pleural friction rub audible at the infarction site
- cyanosis, syncope, and jugular vein distention
- signs of shock (such as weak, rapid pulse and hypotension)

CASE CLIP

Responding to air or amniotic fluid embolism

Ms. G. is a 30-year-old woman in labor and delivery. She had a healthy pregnancy and carried her fetus to 39 weeks' gestation. Her labor and delivery had been uncomplicated, and she was 2 hours postpartum after delivering a healthy 6-pound girl. The nurse entered her room to find her diaphoretic with rapid, shallow breathing. Ms. G. appeared agitated and said she had chills and felt nauseated. Her obstetric pad count had increased over the past hour, and her vaginal output was bright red.

Assessment revealed these vital signs:
- temperature: 99.6° F (37.6° C)
- heart rate (HR): 156 beats/minute
- respiratory rate (RR): 36 breaths/minute
- blood pressure (BP): 76/40 mm Hg
- oxygen saturation: 80% on room air.

On auscultation, the nurse found a grade II/VI systolic ejection murmur at the left sternal border and no S_3. Ms. G.'s breath sounds were diminished at the lung bases bilaterally, but her lungs were otherwise clear. She had diffuse petechiae on her trunk and arms.

The nurse called the rapid response team (RRT). The RRT organized quickly and the nurse responder placed Ms. G. on the monitor/defibrillator and began continuous monitoring of Ms. G.'s heart rate, pulse oximetry, and noninvasive blood pressure. The nurse then proceeded to verify a patent I.V. line and prepared a 1 L bag of I.V. normal saline solution and administered a 500 ml bolus while preparing low dose norepinephrine infusion for hypotension. The respiratory responder immediately placed the patient on a 10 L flow nonrebreather mask and obtained an arterial blood gas sample. Portable chest X-ray and addition laboratory tests were requested by the physician responder along with a request to begin transfer to the intensive care unit (ICU).

The physician responder discussed with the family the need for transfer to the ICU to monitor for possible bleeding disorders and pulmonary complications. Before transfer to the ICU, Ms. G. started to stabilize and had these vital signs:
- HR: 130 beats/minute, following fluid bolus
- RR: 26 breaths/minute
- BP: 96/52 mm Hg, on .02 mcg/kg/minute of norepinephrine
- oxygen saturation: 91% on face mask oxygen.

The arterial blood gas results were: pH 7.49; $PaCO_2$ 19 mm Hg; PaO_2 45 mm Hg; HCO_3^- 31 mEg/L. The portable chest X-ray showed diffuse bilateral pulmonary edema.

Ms. G.'s laboratory tests revealed an increased prothrombin time/partial thromboplastin time, increased D-dimer, and decreased fibrinogen consistent with disseminated intravascular coagulation.

- signs of hypoxia (such as restlessness)
- a right ventricular S_3 gallop audible at the lower sternum
- increased intensity of the pulmonary component of S_2.

Diagnostic tests

These test results can help confirm pulmonary embolism or infarction:

■ Chest X-ray shows a characteristic wedge-shaped infiltrate suggestive of pulmonary embolism. X-rays may rule out other pulmonary diseases and reveal areas of atelectasis, an elevated diaphragm, pleural effusion, and a prominent pulmonary artery.

■ Lung scan shows perfusion defects in areas beyond occluded vessels; a normal lung scan rules out pulmonary embolism.

■ Pulmonary angiography is the most definitive test but poses some risk to the patient (such as allergic reaction to the dye, infection at the catheter site, and kidney failure related to difficulty excreting dye). Its use depends on the uncertainty of the diagnosis and the need to avoid unnecessary anticoagulant therapy (treatment of pulmonary embolism) in high-risk patients.

■ Electrocardiography (ECG) is inconclusive but helps distinguish pulmonary embolism from myocardial infarction. In extensive embolism, ECG may show right axis deviation; right bundle-branch block; tall, peaked P waves; depressed ST segments and T-wave inversions (indicating right heart strain); and supraventricular tachyarrhythmias.

■ Arterial blood gas (ABG) measurements showing decreased partial pressure of arterial oxygen and partial pressure of arterial carbon dioxide are characteristic but don't always occur.

Treatment

Treatment aims to maintain adequate cardiovascular and pulmonary function as the obstruction resolves and to prevent recurrence. Because most emboli resolve within 10 days, treatment consists of oxygen therapy as needed and anticoagulation with heparin to inhibit new thrombus formation.

Patients with massive pulmonary embolism and shock may require thrombolytic therapy with tissue plasminogen activator or streptokinase to enhance fibrinolysis of the pulmonary emboli and remaining thrombi. Hypotension related to pulmonary emboli may be treated with vasopressors.

Treatment for septic emboli requires antibiotic therapy as well as evaluation of the source of infection, particularly in cases of endocarditis. Anticoagulants aren't used to treat septic emboli.

Surgery to interrupt the inferior vena cava is reserved for patients for whom anticoagulants are contraindicated (for example, because of age, recent surgery, or blood dyscrasia) or who have recurrent emboli during anticoagulant therapy. It should be performed only when pulmonary embolism is confirmed by angiography. Surgery consists of vena caval ligation, plication, or insertion of an umbrella filter for blood returning to the heart and lungs. A combination of low-dose

Teaching the patient with pulmonary embolism and infarction

If your patient has pulmonary embolism or infarction, teach him how to use an incentive spirometer to help with deep breathing. Also, warn him not to cross his legs, which can promote thrombus formation.

Most patients need treatment with an oral anticoagulant (such as warfarin [Coumadin]) for 4 to 6 months after a pulmonary embolism. Advise the patient to take the prescribed medication exactly as ordered, to watch for signs of bleeding, and to avoid taking additional medication (even for headaches or colds) or changing medication dosages without consulting his prescriber. Stress the importance of follow-up laboratory tests to monitor anticoagulant therapy. Also encourage family participation in his care.

heparin and dihydroergotamine (Migranal) may be administered to prevent postoperative venous thromboembolism.

Patient care

When caring for a patient with pulmonary embolism, incorporate the following measures into your care plan:
- Give oxygen by nasal cannula or mask.
- Check ABG levels if fresh emboli develop or dyspnea worsens.
- Be prepared to provide equipment for endotracheal intubation and assisted ventilation if breathing is severely compromised. If necessary, prepare to transfer the patient to the intensive care unit according to facility policy.
- Give heparin as ordered by I.V. push or continuous drip.
- Monitor coagulation studies daily and after changes in heparin dosage. Maintain adequate hydration to avoid the risk of hypercoagulability.
- After the patient is stable, encourage him to move about often, and assist with isometric and range-of-motion exercises. Check the temperature and color of his feet to detect venostasis. Never vigorously massage the patient's legs. Ambulate the patient as soon as possible after surgery to prevent venostasis.
- Report frequent pleuritic chest pain so that analgesics can be prescribed.
- Evaluate the patient. His vital signs should be within normal limits, and he should show no signs of bleeding after anticoagulant therapy. (See *Teaching the patient with pulmonary embolism and infarction*.)

Tuberculosis

Tuberculosis (TB) is an acute or chronic infection characterized by pulmonary infiltrates and formation of granulomas with caseation, fibrosis, and cavitation. The American Lung Association estimates that active TB afflicts nearly 7 out of every 100,000 people. The prognosis is excellent with correct treatment.

Causes

Mycobacterium tuberculosis is the major cause of TB. Other strains of mycobacteria may also be involved. Several factors increase the risk of infection, including:
- gastrectomy
- uncontrolled diabetes mellitus
- Hodgkin's lymphoma
- leukemia
- treatment with corticosteroid therapy or immunosuppressant therapy
- silicosis
- human immunodeficiency virus infection.

Pathophysiology

Transmission of TB occurs when an infected person coughs or sneezes, spreading infected droplets. When someone without immunity inhales these droplets, the bacilli are deposited in the lungs.

The immune system responds by sending leukocytes, which initiate an inflammatory response. After a few days, leukocytes are replaced by macrophages.

Bacilli are then ingested by the macrophages and carried off by the lymphatics to the lymph nodes. Then macrophages that ingest the bacilli fuse to form epithelioid cell tubercles (tiny nodules surrounded by lymphocytes). Within the lesion, caseous necrosis develops and scar tissue encapsulates the tubercle. The organism may be killed in the process.

If the tubercles and inflamed nodes rupture, the infection contaminates the surrounding tissue and may spread through the blood and lymphatic circulation to distant sites. This process is called *hematogenous dissemination*.

Assessment

In primary infection, the disease usually doesn't produce symptoms. However, it may produce such nonspecific symptoms as:
- diminished breath sounds and coarse crackles
- fatigue
- weakness
- anorexia
- weight loss
- night sweats
- low-grade fever.

If reinfected, the patient may have:
- cough
- productive mucopurulent sputum
- chest pain.

Patients may also have a latent form of TB which may remain inactive or become active, especially if the immune system is weakened.

Diagnostic tests

Chest X-rays show nodular lesions, patchy infiltrates (many in upper lobes), cavity formation, scar tissue, and calcium deposits. However, they may not distinguish active from inactive TB.

Tuberculin skin tests detect exposure to TB but don't distinguish the disease from uncomplicated infection. Patients from non–North American countries may test positive for TB by skin test due to the positive antibody titer produced by the bacille Calmette-Guérin live vaccine they received as children.

Stains and cultures of sputum, cerebrospinal fluid, urine, drainage from abscess, or pleural fluid show heat-sensitive, nonmotile, aerobic, acid-fast bacilli and confirm the diagnosis.

Treatment

Antitubercular therapy with daily oral doses of isoniazid, rifampin (Rifadin), and pyrazinamide (and sometimes with ethambutol [Myambutol] or streptomycin) for at least 6 months usually cures TB. After 2 to 4 weeks, the disease is typically no longer infectious, and the patient can resume his normal lifestyle while continuing to take medication. A patient with atypical mycobacterial disease or drug-resistant TB may require second-line drugs, such as capreomycin (Capastat), streptomycin, para-aminosalicylic acid, cycloserine (Seromycin), amikacin (Amikin), and fluoroquinolones.

Teaching the patient with TB

To help prevent the spread of tuberculosis (TB), teach a patient in isolation to cough and sneeze into tissues and to dispose of secretions properly. Instruct the patient to wear a mask when he leaves his room. Visitors and staff should wear high-efficiency particulate air respirator masks when in his room.

Remind the patient to get plenty of rest. Stress the need to eat balanced meals, and check the patient's weight weekly.

Teach the signs and symptoms of adverse drug effects, and urge the patient to report them immediately. Emphasize the importance of regular follow-up examinations, and tell the patient to watch for recurring TB.

Advise anyone exposed to an infected patient to receive appropriate diagnostic tests.

Patient care

Your care will focus on preventing the spread of infection as well as providing supportive care. For example:

■ Isolate the infectious patient in a negative-pressure room until he's no longer contagious.

■ Be alert for adverse effects of medications. Pyridoxine (vitamin B_6) is sometimes recommended to prevent peripheral neuropathy caused by large doses of isoniazid. If the patient receives ethambutol, watch for optic neuritis; if it develops, discontinue the drug. Observe for hepatitis and purpura in patients receiving rifampin.

■ Evaluate the patient. His sputum culture should be negative, and secretions should be thin and clear. (See *Teaching the patient with TB.*)

Appendices
Selected references
Audio CD cues:
Heart and breath sounds
Index

Auscultation findings for common cardiovascular disorders

Use this table to review common cardiac disorders and their auscultation findings. Keep in mind that the patient may not have every finding listed for each disorder.

DISORDER	ABNORMAL HEART SOUNDS
Abdominal aortic aneurysm	■ Tachycardia ■ "Blowing" murmur over aorta or "whooshing" sound (bruit)
Aortic insufficiency	■ Early diastolic murmur commonly with midsystolic murmur ■ "Cooing dove" or "musical" diastolic murmur signifies rupture or retroversion of an aortic cusp ■ Diminished A_2 ■ Early ejection click ■ Paradoxical S_2 split ■ S_3–S_4 gallop ■ Soft S_1
Aortic valvular stenosis	■ Midsystolic murmur ■ Paradoxical S_2 split ■ Delayed A_2 and shortened A_2–P_2 interval ■ Aortic ejection sound that radiates widely to neck and along great vessels ■ Systolic ejection sound if not severely stenotic
Atrial septal defect	■ Wide, fixed S_2 split ■ Pulmonic ejection sound ■ Tricuspid component that's louder than mitral component
Cardiac tamponade	■ Muffled or distant heart sounds ■ Pericardial friction rub (with pericarditis)
Cardiogenic shock	■ Gallop rhythm or faint heart sounds ■ Tachycardia
Dilated cardio-myopathy	■ Irregular rhythm (with atrial fibrillation) ■ Pansystolic murmur ■ S_3 and S_4 gallop rhythms
Endocarditis	■ Loud, regurgitant murmur ■ Murmur that changes or appears suddenly, accompanied by fever

DISORDER	ABNORMAL HEART SOUNDS
Heart failure	■ Tachycardia ■ Ventricular gallop (heard over the apex), S_3, or S_4
Hypertrophic obstructive cardiomyopathy	■ Irregular rhythm (with atrial fibrillation) ■ S_3 and S_4 ■ Systolic ejection mumur that becomes louder with Valsalva's maneuver
Mitral insufficiency	■ Holosystolic murmur ■ Decreased S_1 intensity ■ Increased S_2 intensity ■ Accented P_2 ■ S_3 and S_4 gallop ■ Persistent A_2–P_2 splitting during expiration
Mitral stenosis	■ Early and late diastolic murmur (with moderate stenosis) ■ Holodiastolic murmur (in severe stenosis) ■ Loud M_1 ■ Intensified S_1 except with a calcified valve, which produces a soft S_1 ■ Split S_2 ■ Opening snap except with a calcified valve ■ S_3 gallop
Mitral valve prolapse	■ Late systolic or holosystolic murmur ■ Nonejection midsystolic click that's variable in intensity and timing ■ Precordial knock
Myocardial infarction	■ S_3 and S_4 ■ S_1 and S_2 faint and of poor quality ■ Paradoxical splitting of S_2 with left ventricular dysfunction or left bundle-branch block (BBB) ■ Physiologic splitting of S_2 with right BBB, ventricular septal defect, severe mitral insufficiency ■ Harsh holosystolic murmur, crescendo-decrescendo with palpable thrill if ventricular septal rupture
Patent ductus arteriosus	■ Continuous murmur reaching maximum intensity during late systole ■ Murmur envelops S_2 ■ Paradoxical S_2 split ■ Diastolic flow rumble ■ S_3
Pericarditis	■ Pericardial friction rub with both a systolic (loudest) and diastolic component ■ Scratchy, grating, superficial quality
Prosthetic aortic valve	■ Systolic murmur ■ Aortic opening click ■ Aortic closing click ■ Interval between aortic closing click and P_2 that widens during inspiration

DISORDER	ABNORMAL HEART SOUNDS
Prosthetic aortic valve malfunction	■ Long systolic ejection ■ Absent or softened aortic opening click ■ Absent or diminished aortic closing click ■ Diastolic murmur
Prosthetic mitral valve	■ Systolic murmur ■ Mitral closing click ■ Mitral opening click depending on valve type ■ Diastolic murmur depending on valve type
Prosthetic mitral valve malfunction	■ Holosystolic murmur ■ New diastolic murmur or change in intensity or duration of existing one ■ Diastolic rumble ■ Absent mitral closing click
Pulmonary edema	■ S_3 or S_4
Pulmonic insufficiency	■ Early diastolic murmur intensified during inspiration ■ Loud P_2
Pulmonic valve stenosis	■ Midsystolic murmur ■ Systolic ejection click ■ P_2 absent or diminished and delayed ■ Normal or widened S_2 split ■ S_4
Restrictive cardiomyopathy	■ Abnormal or distant heart sounds ■ S_3 or S_4 gallop ■ Systolic murmur
Rheumatic heart disease, rheumatic fever	■ Carditis or valvulitis ■ With carditis, new murmur (usually mitral insufficiency), tachycardia out of proportion to fever, and S_3 gallop ■ With valvulitis, new or changing murmurs and cardiac evidence of heart failure and pericarditis (such as tachycardia, ventricular gallop, and pericardial friction rub)
Supravalvular aortic stenosis	■ Midsystolic murmur ■ Normal S_2 split ■ No aortic ejection sound
Tricuspid stenosis	■ Middiastolic to late-diastolic murmur that increases during inspiration and fades during expiration ■ Normal S_2 or may be split during inspiration ■ Opening snap seldom heard
Ventricular septal defect	■ Loud holosystolic murmur ■ Persistent A_2–P_2 splitting during expiration ■ Abnormal S_3 followed by short, low-frequency, diastolic murmur ■ Pulmonic ejection sound ■ Loud P_2

Auscultation findings for common respiratory disorders

Use this table to review common respiratory disorders and their auscultation findings. Keep in mind that the patient may not have every finding listed for each disorder.

DISORDER	ABNORMAL BREATH SOUNDS
Asbestosis	▪ High-pitched crackles at the end of inspiration ▪ Pleural friction rub
Asthma	▪ Diminished breath sounds ▪ Musical, high-pitched, expiratory polyphonic wheezes ▪ With status asthmaticus, loud and continuous random monophonic wheezes heard, along with prolonged expiration and possible silent chest if severe
Atelectasis	▪ High-pitched, hollow, tubular bronchial breath sounds, crackles, wheezes ▪ Fine, high-pitched, late inspiratory crackles ▪ Bronchophony ▪ Egophony ▪ Whispered pectoriloquy ▪ Inspiratory:expiratory (I:E) ratio: I greater than E over empty lung field
Bronchial stenosis	▪ Loud, continuous, low-pitched, fixed, monophonic wheezes that may disappear in supine position or when turning side to side
Bronchiectasis	▪ Profuse, low-pitched crackles during midinspiration
Chronic bronchitis	▪ Scanty, low-pitched, early inspiratory crackles not affected by position ▪ Loud, musical, high-pitched, expiratory polyphonic wheezes
Chronic obstructive pulmonary disease	▪ Diminished, low-pitched breath sounds ▪ Sonorous or sibilant wheezes ▪ Inaudible bronchophony, egophony, and whispered pectoriloquy ▪ Prolonged expiration ▪ Fine inspiratory crackles
Fibrosing alveolitis	▪ Loud, continuous, high-pitched, sequential wheezes
Interstitial pulmonary fibrosis	▪ Late inspiratory fine crackles not affected by coughing and that may disappear with position change, deep inhalation, or holding of breath ▪ High-pitched bronchial or bronchovesicular breath sounds heard over lower lung regions that are audible through inspiration and expiration ▪ Loud, high-pitched, sequential wheezes of continuous duration ▪ Whispered pectoriloquy

DISORDER	ABNORMAL BREATH SOUNDS
Laryngeal spasm	■ Stridor during inspiration
Pleural effusion	■ Absent or diminished low-pitched breath sounds ■ Occasionally loud bronchial breath sounds ■ Normal breath sounds on contralateral side ■ Bronchophony, egophony, and whispered pectoriloquy at upper border of pleural effusion
Pneumonia	■ High-pitched, tubular bronchial breath sounds heard over affected area during inspiration and expiration ■ Bronchophony ■ Egophony ■ Whispered pectoriloquy ■ Late inspiratory crackles not affected by coughing or position changes ■ I:E ratio 1:1
Pneumothorax	■ Absent or diminished low-pitched breath sounds ■ Inaudible bronchophony, egophony, and whispered pectoriloquy ■ Normal breath sounds on contralateral side
Pulmonary edema	■ Inspiratory and expiratory crackles over the posterior lung bases ■ More profuse crackles and appearance during late inspiration as pulmonary edema worsens ■ Wheezes
Whooping cough	■ Stridor

Selected references

Berman, A., et al. *Kozier & Erb's Fundamentals of Nursing Concepts, Process, and Practice,* 8th ed. Upper Saddle River, N.J.: Prentice Hall Health, 2008.

Bickley, L.S., and Szilagyi, P. *Bates' Guide to Physical Examination and History Taking,* 9th ed. Philadelphia: Lippincott Williams & Wilkins, 2007.

Breath Sounds Made Incredibly Easy. Philadelphia: Lippincott Williams & Wilkins, 2005.

Bursi, F., et al. "Systolic and Diastolic Heart Failure in the Community," *JAMA* 296(18):2209-16, November 2006.

Cardiovascular Care Made Incredibly Visual. Philadelphia: Lippincott Williams & Wilkins, 2007.

Dacey, M.J., et al. "The Effect of a Rapid Response Team on Major Clinical Outcome Measures in a Community Hospital," *Critical Care Medicine* 35(9):2076-82, September 2007.

Ferns, T. "Respiratory Auscultation: How to use a Stethoscope," *Nursing Times* 103(24):28-29, June 2007.

Health Assessment Made Incredibly Visual. Philadelphia: Lippincott Williams & Wilkins, 2007.

Heart Sounds Made Incredibly Easy. Philadelphia: Lippincott Williams & Wilkins, 2005.

Jamison, J.R. *Differential Diagnosis for Primary Care: A Handbook for Healthcare Professionals,* 2nd ed. New York: Churchill Livingstone, 2007.

Kasper, D.L., et al., eds. *Harrison's Principles of Internal Medicine,* 17th ed. New York: McGraw-Hill Book Co., 2008.

Kennedy, S. "Detecting Changes in the Respiratory Status of Ward Patients," *Nursing Standard* 21(49):42-46, August 2007.

McFarlan, S.J., and Hensley, S. "Implementation and Outcomes of a Rapid Response Team," *Journal of Nursing Care Quality* 22(4):314-15; October-December, 2007.

Moore, T. "Respiratory Assessment in Adults," *Nursing Standard* 21(49):48-56, August 2007.

Nurse's 5-Minute Clinical Consult: Signs & Symptoms, Philadelphia: Lippincott Williams & Wilkins, 2007.

Nurse's Quick Check: Diseases, 2nd ed. Philadelphia: Lippincott Williams & Wilkins, 2009.

RN Expert Guides: Cardiovascular Care. Philadelphia: Lippincott Williams & Wilkins, 2008.

RN Expert Guides: Respiratory Care. Philadelphia: Lippincott Williams & Wilkins, 2008.

Shindler, D.M. "Practical Cardiac Auscultation," *Critical Care Nursing Quarterly* 30(2):166-80, April-June 2007.

Smeltzer, S.C., and Bare, B.G. *Brunner and Suddarth's Textbook of Medical-Surgical Nursing,* 11th ed. Philadelphia: Lippincott Williams & Wilkins, 2008.

Tierney, L., et al. *Current Medical Diagnosis and Treatment,* 47th ed. New York: McGraw-Hill Book Co., 2008.

Weinberger, M., and Abu-Hasan, M. "Pseudo-Asthma: When Cough, Wheezing, and Dyspnea are not Asthma," *Pediatrics* 120(4):855-64, October 2007.

Woods, S.L., et al. *Cardiac Nursing,* 5th ed. Philadelphia: Lippincott Williams & Wilkins, 2005.

Audio CD cues:
Heart and breath sounds

Heart sounds

TRACK	SOUND	TRACK	SOUND
1	Normal S_1 and S_2 (base of heart)	21	Summation gallop
2	S_1 (mitral area)	22	Right-sided S_4
3	S_1 split	23	Opening snap of mitral valve
4	Abnormal S_1 split	24	Pulmonic ejection sound
5	Normal S_2 (pulmonic area)	25	Aortic ejection sound
6	S_2 split during inspiration and expirtion	26	Midsystolic click
7	Increased intensity of P_2	27	Innocent systolic ejection murmur
8	Increased intensity of A_2	28	Supravalvular pulmonic stenosis murmur
9	Diminished A_2	29	Pulmonic valvular stenosis murmur
10	Persistent S_2 split during inspiration and expiration	30	Subvalvular pulmonic stenosis murmur
11	Paradoxical S_2 split heard during expiration	31	Supravalvular aortic stenosis murmur
12	Persistent S_2 split	32	Aortic valvular stenosis murmur
13	Persistent S_2 split in pulmonary hypertension	33	Subvalvular aortic stenosis murmur
14	Wide, fixed S_2 split	34	Tricuspid regurgitation (insufficiency) murmur
15	Fused paradoxical S_2 split	35	Holosystolic mitral regurgitation (insufficiency) murmur
16	S_3 over mitral area (S_1, S_2, S_3)	36	Acute mitral regurgitation (insufficiency) murmur
17	Abnormal S_3	37	Mitral valve prolapse murmur with click
18	Pericardial knock	38	Early diastolic aortic regurgitation (insufficiency) murmur
19	Right-sided S_3		
20	S_4 (S_4, S_1, S_2)		

TRACK	SOUND
39	Austin Flint murmur
40	Graham Steell murmur
41	Normal pressure pulmonic valve murmur
42	Mitral stenosis murmur (atrial fibrillation)
43	Mitral stenosis murmur (normal sinus rhythm)
44	Tricuspid stenosis murmur

TRACK	SOUND
45	Cervical venous hum murmur
46	Patent ductus arteriosus murmur
47	Aortic prosthetic valve sound and murmur
48	Mitral prosthetic valve sound and murmur
49	Pericardial friction rub
50	Mediastinal crunch

Breath sounds

TRACK	SOUND
51	Tracheal and mainstem bronchi breath sounds
52	Normal breath sounds over other chest wall areas
53	Bronchovesicular breath sounds
54	Bronchophony (normal)
55	Egophony (normal)
56	Whispered pectoriloquy
57	Tracheal and mainstem bronchi breath sounds
58	Normal breath sounds (midlung)
59	Normal breath sounds (apex)
60	Bronchial breath sounds (consolidation)
61	Bronchial breath sounds (atelectasis)
62	Bronchial breath sounds (fibrosis)
63	Bronchophony (consolidation)
64	Bronchophony (normal)
65	Bronchophony (consolidation)
66	Whispered pectoriloquy (atelectasis)

TRACK	SOUND
67	Whispered pectoriloquy (normal)
68	Egophony (tumor, pleural effusion)
69	Egophony (normal)
70	Diminished breath sounds (shallow breathing)
71	Diminished breath sounds (diaphragmatic paralysis)
72	Absent breath sounds (pneumothorax)
73	Normal breath sounds (pneumothorax)
74	Absent breath sounds (pneumothorax)
75	Diminished breath sounds (pleural effusion)
76	Normal breath sounds (pleural effusion)
77	Diminished breath sounds (pleural effusion)
78	Diminished breath sounds (hyperinflated lungs)
79	Diminished breath sounds (obesity)

Breath sounds (continued)

TRACK	SOUND
80	Diminished breath sounds (positive end-expiratory pressure)
81	Coarse crackles
82	Fine crackles
83	Wheezes
84	Low-pitched wheezes
85	Late inspiratory crackles (atelectasis)
86	Late inspiratory crackles (lobar pneumonia)
87	Late inspiratory crackles (interstitial fibrosis)

TRACK	SOUND
88	Late inspiratory crackles (left ventricular heart failure)
89	Early inspiratory crackles (chronic bronchitis)
90	Early- to mid-inspiratory crackles (bronchiectasis)
91	Pleural crackles
92	Expiratory polyphonic wheezes
93	Fixed monophonic wheezes
94	Sequential inspiratory wheezes
95	Random monophonic wheezes
96	Stridor

Index

i refers to an illustration; t refers to a table.

---

i refers to an illustration; t refers to a table.

---

i refers to an illustration; t refers to a table.

i refers to an illustration; t refers to a table.

i refers to an illustration; t refers to a table.

---

i refers to an illustration; t refers to a table.